PRESCRIPTION
for THE FUTURE

ALSO BY EZEKIEL J. EMANUEL

Healthcare, Guaranteed (2008)

Reinventing American Healthcare (2013)

PRESCRIPTION
for THE FUTURE

The Twelve Transformational Practices
of Highly Effective Medical Organizations

EZEKIEL J. EMANUEL

PUBLICAFFAIRS
New York

Published by PublicAffairs™, an imprint of Perseus Books, LLC,
a subsidiary of Hachette Book Group, Inc.

Library of Congress Cataloging-in-Publication Data is available for this book.
ISBN 978-1-61039-725-4 (HC)
ISBN 978-1-61039-726-1 (EB)

The Hachette Speakers Bureau provides a wide range of authors for speaking events.
To find out more, go to hachettespeakersbureau.com or call 866-376-6591.

Editorial production by Christine Marra, *Marra*thon Production Services.
www.marrathoneditorial.net

Book design by Jane Raese
Set in 11.5-point Albertina

FIRST EDITION
10 9 8 7 6 5 4 3 2 1

DISCLAIMER

The healthcare system is dynamic. In part, this is because of the election of a new administration, its commitment to repealing and replacing the Affordable Care Act without much specific detail, and the consequent uncertainty about what policies will ultimately come out of Washington. This dynamism is partially the result of the ongoing changes currently occurring throughout the healthcare system. Nevertheless, we have reached and exceeded the tipping point of care delivery transformation. Although the direction of change is now clear, the pace at which it will occur in different locales—and whether there might be some temporary setback along the course—remains unclear. For now, all the information is accurate up until the words were set in the book during the spring of 2017.

This book contains many stories. All the patients' names have been changed to protect their privacy. A few physicians' names—such as my primary care physician's name—have been changed, again, to protect their privacy. The names of the physician leaders and executives at the various practices, multispecialty groups, and health systems that I visited as part of my research and case development are real.

Finally, I have several conflicts of interest to disclose. I teach at the University of Pennsylvania and describe some of the innovations at my home institution. Over the years I have given scores of speeches for fees, including at some of the organizations profiled in the book: Kaiser Permanente, Anthem (owner of CareMore), and Advocate Health Care. More importantly, I mention the work of several private, for-profit companies innovating and transforming the system. I work for a venture capital firm, Oak HC/FT, which has investments in 3 of the companies profiled: Aspire, Quartet, and VillageMD: I also sit on the boartd of VillageMD. Oak HC/FT and I have no financial relationship with nor have I received speaking fees or other compensation from other companies and medical organizations profiled in this book, including Aledade, Certify, ChenMed, Dean Clinic, Iora Health, WESTMED, Main Line Oncology, and Hoag Orthopedic Institute.

TO TRUE FRIENDS
WHO HAVE ALWAYS GUIDED ME WISELY

Gregory C. Keating

Corby Kummer

Andrew T. Oram

Henry S. Richardson

Donald Rosenstein

CONTENTS

PRESCRIPTION
for THE FUTURE

INTRODUCTION

Is Exploring Transformation of the
Healthcare System Still Relevant?

W ITH THE ELECTORAL VICTORY of President Donald Trump, it seems reasonable to ask whether this book is still relevant. Have current events overtaken a book advocating reform and transformation of the American healthcare system?

The short answer is no. In fact, the ideas that form the core of this book—ideas aimed at showing how we can develop an innovative, value-driven healthcare delivery system in America—are probably *more* relevant today than ever.

That might seem counterintuitive. Whereas a burst of healthcare reform zeal fueled the 2008 election, the results of the 2016 election can be interpreted as a backlash against the Affordable Care Act (ACA) and the changes it unleashed throughout the healthcare system. Indeed, Republicans' most explicit and fundamental battle cry during the 2016 election was "repeal and replace." To some degree their victory hinged on their pledge to dismantle Obamacare. Many people might logically deduce that further efforts to transform the delivery of American healthcare are misguided and mistaken.

Wrong. Reforming the healthcare system is about more than just the latest battle over the ACA or any particular healthcare regulation. Two fundamental problems plague the American healthcare system: (1) it underperforms on almost every conceivable metric, and (2) the public, small businesses, corporations, and governments all find it unaffordable. Improving the American healthcare system is something every patient, every small business owner, every corporate executive, every physician, nurse, and other practitioner, every politician and policy-maker should care about. The system desperately needs to be fixed.

This book is a transformation manual, a guide to updating the health system's core: caring for patients both sick and healthy. It will help medical organizations that want to transform their care but need guidance on the right steps to take and the right sequence in which to take them.

No matter how you measure it, the American healthcare system continues to underperform. Tens of millions of people are still uninsured. Health expenditures remain astronomically high—27% higher per capita than the next highest spending country, Luxembourg. Despite these exorbitant expenditures, health outcomes in the United States are not 27%, 10%, or even 5% better than in other developed countries. Although we arguably exceed the rest of the world in a few health outcomes—and even these are contentiously debated—such as cancer survival, trauma, and organ transplantation, we lag behind in most health and healthcare domains. On even some basic measures of health system quality—life expectancy, infant and youth mortality, immunization rates, behavioral health, asthma survival, and control of diabetes—the United States falls well below other developed countries. And there are endless complaints about impersonal care, hospital-acquired infections, rushed office visits, excessive admissions to the ICU, and too many high-tech interventions at the end of life. Such inconsistent and relatively poor performance at such a high cost should infuriate any responsible corporate executive. It rightfully infuriates the American public.

Unfortunately, this underperformance is nothing new. It did not begin with the ACA. In fact, the ACA narrowed the gap. Since its enactment in 2010, 22 million Americans have become insured, healthcare cost growth has slowed to an historic low, and by modestly reducing hospital readmissions, hospital-acquired infections, and other preventable errors, quality has improved.

Nevertheless, the public remains unconvinced that the ACA has improved the situation. Ironically, polls reveal that the public likes much of what the ACA enacted—the no preexisting disease exclusion, allowing young adults to be on their parents' health insurance plans until age 26, no annual or lifetime limits on insurance coverage, limits on insurance company profits, coverage of preventive services without deductibles, and subsidies to buy private insurance. Yet the ACA became a scapegoat, the nidus for all Americans' lingering anger about the healthcare system.

Today Americans are primarily angry about the affordability of health insurance and healthcare. Drug costs have skyrocketed, as epitomized by the 56-fold price increase for Daraprim by Turing Pharmaceuticals, the $600 for EpiPens, and $1,000 per pill for the hepatitis C drug Sovaldi. A visit to the emergency room, even for something as simple as a few stitches, can cost $5,000 or more. And insurance premiums have increased for most consumers while their plans have grown skimpier with ever-shrinking networks and ever-increasing deductibles. Although coverage gaps and preexisting condition exclusions were the big concerns in 2008, today the public is demanding reforms that focus on *affordability*.

The American healthcare system thus remains ripe for transformation. While some fret that the uncertainty surrounding the Trump administration's desire to repeal and replace the ACA will stifle innovation, that uncertainty is ultimately transitory. The system's underperformance and excessive costs are fundamental and structural. After the rhetoric and heat of the moment dissipate, addressing these issues will re-emerge as the primary locus of concern. Fundamentals provide the surest foundation to weather the vicissitudes of uncertainty.

Rather than focusing on the latest rumor about repeal and replace or the ups and downs of Washington political maneuvering, it is prudent to aim for what will necessarily be important both 5 and 10 years from now. For healthcare, that means achieving high-value care. That is where the system is ultimately headed. And that is where smart money, lots of it from venture capital and private equity, is investing. Although there may be some twists and turns off a direct course, high-value care is the eventual destination. That is where the best medical organizations are also headed. They are not, like inexperienced hockey players, converging on the puck but, like seasoned pros, skating to where the puck will be. Although there are many medical organizations currently making healthy profits who are skeptical of the need for change and resistant to innovating in the delivery of care, as the system evolves they will become less and less relevant, the Kodaks of healthcare.

The only way to simultaneously address the underperformance and unaffordability of the system is to transform care delivery. To address underperformance, we must improve the quality of care and out-comes—reduce preventable complications and errors, ensure patients are consistently prescribed the right tests and treatments, and create support networks and systems to ensure they actually adhere to them. This can only be done by transforming how physicians, hospitals, and other providers deliver care.

To address unaffordability, we must sustainably moderate health-care cost increases—keep per person healthcare cost increases to no more than growth in the GDP. This requires eliminating waste in the widest sense—namely, eliminating unnecessary services that do not improve health yet increase costs, reducing the per-unit cost of deliv-ering each medical service, and prescribing lower-cost but clinically equivalent services. This too can only be achieved through delivery system transformation.

Transformation does not happen spontaneously. It requires the right financial, legal, and practice environment to occur. Fortunately many of these factors were introduced by the ACA and are likely to live on given their general lack of public controversy. First, even as payment re-mains largely fee-for-service, the system is inexorably moving toward alternative payment models such as bundled payments and capita-tion. This transition has incentivized physicians, hospitals, and other healthcare providers to start delivering higher-value care. Second, the ACA introduced accountable care organizations (ACOs), the Center for Medicare and Medicaid Innovation, and policies penalizing hospitals that have high rates of readmission and hospital-acquired infections. These reforms, along with the bundled payment experiments, re-inforce and amplify the drive to transform care delivery. Finally, in late 2015 Congress enacted the Medicare Access and CHIP Reauthorization Act—better known as MACRA—that institutionalized the govern-ment's drive to change how it pays for care while further encouraging physicians to adopt alternative payment schemes. This combination of policy changes has pushed the American healthcare system past the tipping point on transformation. The genie is out of the bottle; there is no turning back now.

Importantly, the reforms created by the ACA are necessary but not sufficient for transformation. The critical next step is for physicians, hospitals, and other healthcare providers to comprehensively rethink the processes of care delivery—from simple processes like scheduling office visits and rooming patients to more complex clinical decision-making processes like building out standardized care protocols, implementing effective chronic care coordination, and integrating behavioral health services into routine office flows. This book is meant to help medical organizations that want to be in the right place in the near future—near the high-value puck—focus their energies on the right issues and change their practices in the best ways.

The case studies in this book portray medical organizations that are transforming how they deliver care to improve quality and patient experience while simultaneously lowering costs. Delineating these practices will also help physicians and hospitals transform their practices to deliver higher-value care. Lastly, the insights about transformation can help Americans choose better physicians and practices for their own care.

This book aims to nudge—even push—medical organizations toward that better delivery system. It shows how, by adopting the 12 transformational practices delineated in Chapters 4, 5 and 6, physician practices and health systems can get there.

Finally, this book offers enduring advice to practitioners that is not tied to any particular piece of governmental legislation or regulation or to any debate among politicians about healthcare proposals. One election or one more piece of legislation does not render irrelevant the guidance about how to transform the delivery of care to patients. Although the next few years may be rocky, the American healthcare system will ultimately become better performing and more affordable in the long run. This book provides lasting insights for medical organizations on how to realize those goals and consistently improve care and patient experience while controlling healthcare costs. Its advice will not go out of style or be superseded by any particular election or the vagaries of Washington; indeed, the case studies, transformational practices, and lessons in this book will help position medical organizations for the future regardless of the momentary vicissitudes created by the 2016 election and related political upheavals.

Chapter 1

FAILING MISS HARRIS

IT WAS A HOT SUMMER DAY in 2014 when, suddenly, Miss Paige Harris passed out in her sister's living room. Her sister called an ambulance, which rushed her to Mercy Philadelphia Hospital a few blocks away. The emergency room physicians determined she had suffered neither a heart attack nor a stroke and diagnosed her with sick sinus syndrome, which intermittently prevents normal electrical impulses from going throughout her heart and beginning the process of pumping blood. The ER physicians transferred Miss Harris to an affiliated hospital, Mercy Fitzgerald Hospital, where a cardiologist placed an automatic implantable cardioverter defibrillator (AICD) in her chest. The AICD serves as both a pacemaker, electrically stimulating Miss Harris's heart if it is beating too slowly, and a defibrillator, shocking her heart if it stops beating altogether. Yet Miss Harris is confused about the AICD. She calls it a pacemaker, yet she cannot describe what it actually does. She cannot recall anyone asking her for consent but does not believe she could have refused the procedure.

Miss Harris, in her full-length, pink zip-up dressing gown and black do-rag, is an adorable 95-year-old African American woman who, because she is stooped over, looks even smaller than her 5-feet-1 height would suggest. She has a lovely open face that always seems to be smiling, even when she is describing her pains and the frustrations of managing her medications and physician appointments. Her living room has a large TV pushed up against one wall, with a few pictures and knick-knacks decorating the other walls. One piece of artwork is a particularly striking blue primativist picture of a church interior, with 2 dried-out palm fronds draping the frame.

Miss Harris has a long history of high blood pressure and congestive heart failure, leading to severe shortness of breath. Consequently, she sits most of the time: "Anything I do now is hard work." Most days Miss Harris simply sits in an easy chair a few feet from the TV; the chair electrically tilts forward when she wants to get up. Game shows or gospel music play in the background, keeping Miss Harris company as she works her way through thick word-search puzzle books. She shuffles around her small living room–dining room area with a walker.

After her fainting spell Miss Harris moved in with her 93-year-old sister, Mrs. Lilly Johnson, because her shortness of breath made it too difficult to care for herself. At first, Mrs. Johnson did all the housework and helped Miss Harris bathe, dress, and climb the stairs. Six months ago, however, Mrs. Johnson was diagnosed with gastric cancer. Standing in her purple blouse and jeans, Mrs. Johnson appears energetic, but upon closer inspection one can tell that the cancer is taking its toll. The numerous skin folds on her arms attest to the weight and muscle mass she has lost. Mrs. Johnson no longer has the strength to help Miss Harris up the stairs to use the house's 1 restroom located on the 2nd floor or to take a bath. Instead, when Miss Harris needs to use the restroom or go up to bed at the end of the day, she maneuvers her walker to the bottom of the stairs, clutches the bannister, then crawls like a toddler on all fours up the 14 stairs. This self-reliance has been difficult: she is unsteady on her feet, and 2 months ago she fell while getting into the bath. Fortunately she did not break anything, but this episode left Miss Harris fearful. She has not bathed since, instead settling for washing herself off in the sink. Obviously what would be most helpful for Miss Harris is not her high-technology AICD or an office visit to her board-certified cardiologist but rather an aide who could help her climb the stairs and help her bathe.

Miss Harris hardly ever goes outside. She often feels sad and frustrated that she cannot go to the local Sharon Baptist Church. This is at least somewhat alleviated by monthly visits in her home from a church member. A few women from the church also bring Miss Harris sermons recorded on a DVD, an act that Miss Harris is grateful for: "It's not the same as being there, but I do like hearing the sermon."

As Miss Harris describes her situation, sadness clouds her face and her eyes begin to well up:

I'm no good to myself and nobody else. Can't do nothing for myself. Lilly's [Mrs. Johnson's] sick herself, and I'm a burden on her. I can't do nothing I want to do. I don't want to be a burden to her. Lilly says I'm not a burden, but I don't want her to do my washing and everything. I've always been independent. Always been the one helping everyone else. Now I can't do nothing for myself. I don't want to burden her.

Miss Harris then begins to talk about her wishes: "I want to be comfortable. But I'm ready, I'm ready ever since I had my heart attack. Ready whenever the Good Lord is ready to do His work."

After her discharge from the hospital a visiting nurse was assigned to check in on Miss Harris once a week. Surprisingly, after 2 years the visiting nurse, Trina, still comes once a week. Trina's tasks mostly involve taking Miss Harris's blood pressure and weight along with filling all 28 compartments in her plastic pill organizer to ensure Miss Harris has all her medications for the week. This includes vitamins, minerals, and 10 different prescription medications, amounting to 19 pills each and every day. In the 2 years since her fainting episode, Miss Harris has avoided any hospital admission, though she did go to the ER once for abdominal pain that was diagnosed as a urinary tract infection and was treated with antibiotics.

One of the few things Miss Harris still looks forward to are her monthly visits from McKenzie, a nurse practitioner (NP) from a palliative care company called Aspire. Aspire specializes in providing home care for patients who are not yet in the last 6 months of life, at which point they might qualify for hospice. Using a predictive algorithim, Cigna, her Medicare Advantage managed-care company, identified Miss Harris for palliative care. Although Miss Harris did not exhibit many of the "red flags" Cigna uses to identify the terminally ill, such as repeated hospitalizations or having cancer, she is a frail 95-year-old with serious congestive heart failure and qualified by the more qualitative metric often used by Aspire: "Is she a patient that you would not be surprised to see die within the next 12 months?" For Miss Harris the answer was "yes," and so, about 1 year ago, they assigned McKenzie to her.

When McKenzie arrives for her monthly visit Miss Harris's face lights up in a smile. And throughout McKenzie's visit Miss Harris repeatedly asks, "You ain't going to stop coming?" McKenzie always promises that she will not. When reassured, Miss Harris responds, "Oh good. I'd have a fit if you stop coming."

One of the initial things McKenzie did when she first met Miss Harris was to talk about her end-of-life care wishes. Miss Harris made it pretty clear that she did not want to go back to the hospital or get anything "new" done, proclaiming that "If my heart stops, I don't want to change it." When pressed, Miss Harris openly states her preferences: Resuscitation? "No." Being put on a ventilator? "No." Dialysis? "No." Hydration and artificial nutrition? "No. I only want comfort measures, and certainly not the intensive care unit."

McKenzie helped Miss Harris document her wishes by filling out a Physicians Orders for Life-Sustaining Treatment (POLST) form—a kind of expanded Do Not Resuscitate Order. The two also filled out an Advance Care Directive appointing Mrs. Johnson as her power of attorney for these healthcare choices. Miss Harris keeps these forms right on her smoky-gray glass dining room table. As she talks, Miss Harris runs her fingers over them, almost as if she is caressing a rosary. When McKenzie asks whether the forms should be kept somewhere safer, Miss Harris insists that the dining table in the house's main room is fine—it is the best place to ensure the forms' availability should anything happen.

When asked whether there is anything she wants to do before she dies, Miss Harris says, "I'd love to see my great-nephew grow up. I want him to graduate high school, go to college, and make something of himself. I didn't finish school. Wish I'd gone back to school, so I always tell him to go to college. Don't put off going." If she could see that, Miss Harris explains, "then I would be ready for God to do what He wants to do."

McKenzie has tried to get Miss Harris additional assistance to help her cook meals and bathe. But even for an educated, health-literate nurse practitioner, the process of applying for Miss Harris's home assistance has been tortuous. A few months ago, McKenzie and Miss Harris filled out the extensive paperwork necessary to apply for a home aide. Weeks passed, yet they heard nothing. Finally, someone from the Department of Public Welfare came out and evaluated Miss Harris's needs. The official was certain that Miss Harris would qualify but said it would take at least 2 more weeks for the paperwork to be processed and approved and then probably a few more weeks to schedule an aide to start coming to help Miss Harris at home. Yet even after this visit another set of papers was sent to Miss Harris from the Department of Public Welfare. This 11-page document was to assess Miss Harris's assets in order to ensure she qualifies for, as they called it, "County Assistance, Medicaid or Long Term Care." She did. The process has, in short, been both confusing and frustratingly inefficient for McKenzie.

During one visit McKenzie weighs Miss Harris—no increase to indicate worsening congestive heart failure—and notes that her breathing is clear and that oxygenation of her blood is normal. Although Miss Harris's blood pressure is elevated, this is not that unusual. Still, McKenzie arranges for Trina to retake Miss Harris's blood pressure early the following week to make sure nothing is amiss. McKenzie also reviews the pill organizer to see if Miss Harris is taking her medications properly. The pills seem poorly organized, and the day's bedtime pill container is unexpectedly empty. "I have them pills in my pocket," Miss Harris explains, and she pulls out of her pink dressing gown a small wad of tissue tied together with a black rubber band. She opens the tissue packet to show McKenzie the 3 pills, explaining, "That way I'm sure I have the pills when I go up and lay down at night." McKenzie notices that one pill bottle is empty, so she calls the pharmacy to make sure it is refilled and sent to Miss Harris's home.

Then Miss Harris complains about pain, moving her hand to the right side of her chest. Although the dull pain is pretty constant, Miss Harris notes that, "It's not getting any worse." She seems to think it is related to going up and down the stairs, as holding onto the bannister strains her shoulder. McKenzie asks whether Miss Harris is still doing her physical therapy, so she demonstrates the physical therapy exercises for her right shoulder, saying, "Forty times I do them. Three times a day." To help cope with the pain, McKenzie also suggests using a pain-relief cream like Icy Hot.

As she talks, Miss Harris fingers through a stack of small medical appointment cards. Her old primary care physician has recently retired. When asked about her new primary care physician—who, fortunately, visits her in her home—Miss Harris says, "I don't know. She came, asked questions, filled out paperwork, and left." On October 26 she has an appointment with a nephrologist, and before that appointment she must fill out a form because the doctor wants her to get urine and blood tests. On November 2 Miss Harris has an appointment with the cardiologist who put in her AICD.

Her physician appointments are the only time Miss Harris goes outside, and each visit is a major undertaking:

> I got to see if anybody nearby who has a car can drive me. But it's hard to get anyone who's free in the daytime. And I got to pay them to drive me... . There [at the appointment] I always got to go around to one place for the sheet, I got to go to another place for the test, and another for the doctor.

Her sister, standing next to Miss Harris, chimes in that her experience is significantly better than what Miss Harris goes through at Mercy:

> I love it at Presbyterian [Hospital] 'cause there they got it organized. I only got to go to one place to register, and then they bring me back and do all the blood work and doctor visits in one place. I don't have to move around. Plus, with cancer they bring me, I don't have to get someone to drive me there.

When asked why she is going to the kidney doctor and what the blood and urine tests are for, Miss Harris says she doesn't know. Similarly, she is not sure why the cardiologist needs to check out her defibrillator, as it has not gone off and she has not fainted. And it is obvious from her voice and body language that Miss Harris is dreading all the effort it will take to make the arrangements she will need for each visit—asking the neighbors to drive her and moving around the hospital for the tests and office visit. But these appointments are scheduled, and she seems to think she must go. She wants to be a "good patient." Indeed, as a frail, kindly, elderly woman without a high school diploma or much health literacy, she hardly seems like the type of patient who would question a physician's recommendation, and certainly not for something he claimed was necessary to keep her heart beating or make sure her kidneys were working properly.

IN MANY WAYS Miss Harris is lucky. She is part of Independence-at-Home, a program that has primary care physicians conduct visits for frail, elderly patients in their homes instead of an office; she has a visiting nurse who comes and refills her pill organizer to ensure she is compliant with her medications; and she has a palliative care nurse practitioner who sees her every month and, more importantly, has gone over—and documented—her end-of-life care wishes in official forms that are readily available. Hopefully, if something goes wrong—should Miss Harris lose consciousness or have some other acute medical event—these forms will prevent her from being resuscitated and rushed to the hospital and into the ICU, where she does not want to be.

Too few frail, elderly patients actually receive these benefits.

But Miss Harris also illustrates the failings of the American healthcare system. She is subject to a fragmented system, one that lacks coordination and clear care plans and frequently deviates from or even ignores patients' wishes—especially when those wishes are to do as little as possible. Despite being a 95-year-old with serious congestive heart failure and renal failure, Miss Harris ended up with an AICD, which costs, depending upon the hospital, between $30,000 and $55,000 to put in. Even worse, it is unclear whether Miss Harris even wanted the AICD to begin with.

In the 2 years since, Miss Harris acquired 6 healthcare providers: 4 physicians—a primary care physician, a nephrologist, a cardiologist for the ACID, and a "regular" cardiologist—along with a visiting nurse and a visiting palliative care nurse practitioner. None of these providers share a common electronic medical record or a common care plan. The providers do not huddle—or even get on a conference call—once a month to update one another. Miss Harris is taking 19 pills a day, yet no physician or pharmacist has reviewed them or taken her through a systematic "demedication" process to see whether she can take fewer pills; instead, the physicians frequently seem to be adding another pill.

Every 3 months Miss Harris has to go in to see at least one specialist, a trip that always requires major effort—and costs her money, as she must pay a neighbor to drive her. It is unclear both *why* Miss Harris needs to see these specialists and what *specifically* they are doing to help her. Mostly the specialists appear to be attending to their single organ system without ever stopping to consider how their care fits into the larger picture that is Miss Harris. For example, Miss Harris has made it clear that if her kidneys continue to fail, she does not want dialysis. Miss Harris's primary care physician is perfectly capable of monitoring her blood pressure and kidney function. So why must she even see a nephrologist? There is little coordination between the primary care physician and the nephrologist. And what is the cardiologist for? Miss Harris has a "do not resuscitate" order. It is unclear whether she ever actually, voluntarily consented to the AICD in the first place, and it remains unclear why it has not been turned off. Still, Miss Harris dutifully goes every 3 months to see her cardiologist because he says he needs to be sure the machine is "working."

None of her physicians seems to have taken a step back and asked critical questions like: What are we doing for Miss Harris? What is the medical and, more importantly, life purpose guiding the tests and prescriptions we order? What does Miss Harris want? Should all visits to the nephrologist and cardiologist be canceled?

What Miss Harris really needs is not another appointment with a highly trained, board-certified medical specialist, but simply an aide to come to her house and help her bathe. Unfortunately, that is outside the scope of the medical system—it is in the social service system—and takes several packets of multipage forms, a home assessment, and weeks of waiting to obtain.

Each of Miss Harris's individual medical services—the implantable cardiac defibrillator, the blood tests, the physical therapy, the pills, the home visits, the palliative care planning—may be done well. It is obvious that her providers are carefully and regularly monitoring Miss Harris's medication compliance, weight, oxygenation, blood pressure, renal function, painful shoulder, and other physiological parameters—and intervening if necessary.

Yet it is also equally obvious that the system is failing. Miss Harris gets fragmented care from 6 largely uncoordinated providers. She often receives unnecessary—low- or no-value—care as a result of regularly seeing physicians she does not need to see; undergoing tests that, even if seriously abnormal, would never alter her care; and receiving medical interventions she does not want. Yet despite this mountain of care Miss Harris does not have the few—and cheap—services that would help her with bathing and the other activities of daily life and would truly improve her quality of life.

Who knows how much all of this uncoordinated, unnecessary medical care is costing—certainly thousands of dollars per year and, during the year that Miss Harris received the AICD, tens of thousands of dollars. Maybe her Advance Care Directive and POLST form will preempt additional tens of thousands of dollars spent on an ambulance, emergency room assessments, and ICU stays at the very end of her life. Then again, maybe not.

COULD THE American healthcare system do a better job of caring for Miss Harris? The answer is most certainly yes.

But that is not the critical question. Instead, we must ask: How should the healthcare system transform to ensure that the millions of Miss Harrises in the country—indeed, all Americans—receive consistently higher-quality and lower-cost care? The other critical question is: How can the Miss Harrises of the country—and their concerned and caring relatives—distinguish a good medical practice from a poor one?

This book is about that transformation in the delivery of care in the United States. It explores different parts of the healthcare system that have transformed the way they care for patients to achieve higher-quality, more patient-focused, and lower-cost care.

For this book I did not study the healthcare systems whose names everyone seems to know, who many assume to be the "best" and most transformed—systems like the Mayo Clinic, the Cleveland Clinic, Intermountain Healthcare, and so on. Instead, I studied small physician offices and large multispecialty group practices, accountable care organizations, large managed-care organizations, and even for-profit companies, all of whom are transforming care largely under the radar. Some are household names, and some are known within the health policy community, but many are relatively unknown even to physicians and health policy experts. Admittedly, I have not selected the practices or organizations in any systematic, quantitative manner but rather in a careful, if somewhat haphazard, way. I heard about one great practice or healthcare system and decided to see if it had transformational practices that others could learn from. I attended a lecture by someone who transformed some aspect of his or her practice, and then I studied those changes. I was asked to speak somewhere and determined that their processes of care were worth examining. Undoubtedly, there are myriad other practices and health systems throughout the United States that are doing impressive work and should also be studied, characterized, and celebrated for their innovations in improving patient care.

The practices and systems I studied admit that they are in the process—not the culmination—of transformation. They are still experimenting, learning from their mistakes, and refining their approaches. Indeed, none of the medical organizations have implemented all 12 of the transformational practices I have identified, nor are they necessarily succeeding in all dimensions of care transformation. Nevertheless, each practice and group included in this book is innovating in particular ways we all can and should learn from as we try to improve the delivery of care in the United States.

This is a qualitative book based on case studies. I have relied largely on stories of transformation. It is a book that looks at particular cases—the people who are driving change and the specific transformations they have instituted. Much of this book is based on what qualitative researchers call "saturation"—carefully observing and ascribing significance when various diverse groups and organizations, in many different geographic locations, are independently reporting similar things. I saw this with chronic care management, for example, as multiple groups, working independently, were basically arriving at the same conclusion about this practice: they must not outsource care management but rather co-locate a chronic care manager in the physician's office to ensure proper coordination of care for high-risk, high-cost patients. The care manager develops a personal, face-to-face relationship with patients and then sees and calls the patients frequently to ensure they are doing well. Chronic care managers meet with the other team members weekly or monthly to formally discuss and update the care plans and interventions needed to keep the patients healthy and out of the emergency room and hospital. Every organization that has transformed care management has done it pretty much this same way.

Even though the practices were selected in a haphazard way using qualitative methods, I have attempted to systematically delineate the key components of each of the 12 transformational practices of care as well as of other practices that are frequently touted as beneficial, but rarely prove effective or pivotal to transformation. Interestingly, no single practice, multispecialty group, or health system I visited and studied has implemented all 12 transformational practices. Many have made significant—double-digit—improvements in quality, patient experience, and cost, and still have room to improve.

Although this book does not claim or seek to be a comprehensive study of all—or even necessarily the very best—transformed practices and healthcare organizations in the United States, I hope this framework will offer other physician practices and medical organizations guidance on how they can change their processes of care. I am not claiming to have the end-all answer to transforming American healthcare; rather, as I have said before, the 12 practices in this book are a productive place to start.

The aim of this book is not to decree that every medical organization in the United States must implement all 12 transformational practices; rather, it is to encourage all practices, health systems, accountable care organizations, and multispecialty groups to begin to put these transformational practices into action. My hope is that by describing these practices and how different physician groups and health systems have implemented them, hundreds of thousands of others around the country that want—and need—to change will have a roadmap with major landmarks, useful examples, and even places to turn for guidance.

Although Miss Harris's story is sobering, maybe even frustrating and depressing, this is an optimistic book. Today there is the potential for truly positive, groundbreaking change in the American healthcare system—more so than at any other time since the 1910 publication of the Flexner Report. Change is happening on a relatively small scale but in a multitude of places. Yet change has not yet coalesced, so it can be hard for many people to see and feel its effects—hard to distinguish the signal from the noise. But the signals regarding the transformational practices necessary to improve patient care and control costs are beginning to emerge. This book tries to identify—and systematize—those signals so they can be detected, copied, further refined, and spread even further.

This book is not only for physicians, nurses, hospital administrators, consultants, and others working in the healthcare system. I hope that it will give every patient the tools to begin to recognize the strengths or failings of any healthcare service they encounter. Chapter 9 will help average Americans like Miss Harris—or, more likely, her relatives—apply the 12 transformational practices in choosing the physician and healthcare organization that will deliver to them much better and more patient focused care.

That transformation of care for patients like Miss Harris is not only possible, but even inevitable, begins with the changes that have taken place in the policy landscape starting with the Affordable Care Act—Obamacare. These changes, and in particular changes in the way physicians and hospitals are paid and made to report on their quality, are necessary parts of the foundation for transforming patient care. That is the subject of the next chapter, which will show the groundwork that must be laid to begin to shift toward high-value care.

Chapter 2

THE STIMULUS
FOR CHANGE

The ACA, Bundled Payments,
MACRA, and Beyond

T HE AMERICAN healthcare system is currently undergoing its most significant change in over a century. In 1910 Abraham Flexner published his eponymous report that began the process of transforming medical training in the United States and Canada. It condemned numerous proprietary, for-profit medical schools run by practitioners who offered short training programs, usually with no educational prerequisites. The Flexner Report advocated instead for university-affiliated medical schools with classes taught by university-appointed medical professors. These schools would require students to be high school graduates, have a prerequisite of multiple years of college-level basic science training that would be followed by 2 years of preclinical coursework as well as 2 years of hospital-based clinical training. The Flexner Report exposed the dire need for higher rigor and standards in physician training and ended the state of complacency that had plagued the medical academy. Its basic model still shapes medical education. Today's emerging transformation of the delivery of care will be similarly momentous.

What the Flexner Report did for medical education the Affordable Care Act (ACA) of 2010 and the Medicare Access and CHIP Reauthorization Act (MACRA) of 2015 will do for healthcare delivery. Regardless of whether these laws remain on the books, they mark an irreversible turning point in American health policy. They acknowledge the century's long, unsustainable, fragmented, fee-for-service system and initiated its widespread demise. More importantly, they began a concerted shift toward policies that encourage the delivery of higher-value care.

For decades many leaders in medicine, most politicians, and a large majority of the American public insisted that the United States had the best healthcare system in the world. They pointed to the numerous venerable hospitals in the United States, such as the Mayo Clinic, Massachusetts General Hospital, Cleveland Clinic, and Johns Hopkins Hospital, as well as to internationally leading biomedical research institutions like the National Institutes of Health (NIH), Harvard Medical School, University of California San Francisco (UCSF), and Rockefeller University. But in the later 2000s, as the debate around healthcare reform intensified, it became increasingly clear that regardless of these exemplars of medical care and research, the larger American healthcare system was underperforming by almost every measure.

Prior to passage of the ACA, Americans' access to healthcare was inadequate. Nearly 50 million Americans were uninsured, and millions more were underinsured, with austere, unreliable policies that failed to protect them from grave financial loss or bankruptcy if they developed a serious illness. An additional problem was the healthcare system's persistently high cost. Spending over $2.6 trillion in 2010, the US healthcare system constituted the 5th largest economy in the world, just smaller than the entire German economy. In 2010 the per capita costs were nearly $8,402.

Despite such huge expenditures, healthcare quality was haphazard at best. Even if there were pockets of greatness, the United States as a whole performed poorly on numerous indicators, such as life expectancy, infant mortality, immunization rates, blood pressure control, and deaths from hospital-acquired infections. Embarrassingly, the US healthcare system had a relatively low World Health Organization (WHO) ranking: 37th globally in 2010, behind countries like Cyprus, Greece, and Morocco. Even if this precise ranking was inaccurate, it nonetheless indicated that there were legitimate issues plaguing the American system. It degraded the claim that the United States had "the best healthcare system in the world."

Why was the US healthcare system underperforming? A consensus emerged among both conservative and liberal health-policy experts that there were 2 fundamental defects causing both the cost and quality problems. First, the fee-for-service payment system for physicians and hospitals rewarded the wrong actions—like putting an AICD into Miss Harris when she is "ready for God" and wanted no life-sustaining treatments. Fee-for-service payment made expensive hospitalizations and surgical procedures financially lucrative for hospitals. It encouraged clinicians to do more tests and procedures while ignoring the costs when ordering them. Additionally, fee-for-service paid the same amount regardless of the quality of care or its medical appropriateness. Even worse, fee-for-service incentivized treating people only when they presented with an illness; it did not encourage keeping people healthy in the first place.

Fee-for-service also fragments care. By paying physicians and hospitals separately, there is no financial incentive for them to work together and coordinate patient care. This may even be an incentive not to collaborate. Consequently patients like Miss Harris often see both a primary care physician and a nephrologist, even though her primary care physician could competently monitor her kidney function. Similarly, patients are frequently admitted and discharged from hospitals without their primary care physician even being informed, which hampers timely follow-up and increases the chances that they will be re-admitted within 30 days.

The second fundamental defect was that the system discouraged physicians and hospitals from systematically measuring, reporting on, and improving the quality of their care. Indeed, by receiving additional payments for every treatment associated with a hospital-acquired infection or readmission for congestive heart failure, hospitals had an incentivize to disregard many dimensions of quality. Moreover, without rigorous performance data and objective benchmarks, it was impossible to create effective programs to improve quality.

Two fundamental changes were needed to create the environment that would enable transforming the American healthcare system to one focused on keeping people healthy, improving quality, and lowering costs. First, there needed to be a shift away from fee-for-service to so-called alternative payment systems that reward physicians and hospitals for delivering higher-value care. Second, assessments and reporting of physicians' and hospitals' quality needed to become routine.

The ACA began a process of instituting these 2 fundamental reforms.

THE AFFORDABLE CARE ACT
ENABLES TRANSFORMATION

The ACA may be the most significant American healthcare reform in a century. The Act signaled that business would not continue as usual and that the American healthcare system would undergo a seismic transformation. Indeed, the ACA's most important legacy is not any particular provision but rather how it changed the psychology of all the people involved in the provision of healthcare—the physicians and nurses, hospital administrators and insurance company executives, home health owners and skilled nursing facilities owners. And this change in psychology will not easily be undone even with "repeal and replace." Unlike any particular provision related to the mandate or insurance exchanges, this change in attitude is permanent.

Conventional wisdom holds that the ACA was 2,000 or more pages and that 90% of it addressed increasing access to insurance. This assertion is wrong on both counts. The ACA encompasses 10 "titles" and only 906 pages, but only 2 titles, comprising about 225 pages, address the health insurance exchanges, subsidies, and the expansion of Medicaid. While they have drawn the most public attention and debate and had the immediate impact of expanding coverage to about 22 million Americans, these titles represent only a small portion of the law and its impact.

In fact, the ACA has done much more. It contains numerous provisions aimed at changing how physicians, hospitals, and other providers are paid and how patients are cared for. These reforms, though significant, have received far less public attention. That is understandable. These reforms are embodied in complex regulatory details that are of interest mainly to hospitals, physicians, skilled nursing facilities, durable medical equipment supply companies, and other providers who receive government reimbursement. Despite their obscurity, these reforms are fundamentally important because they encourage providers to change how they actually care for Americans like Miss Harris.

The ACA contains at least 9 different provisions that accelerated this budding revolution (see Table 2.1, page 214). To understand the nature and scope of the changes the ACA induced, it is worth briefly highlighting a few of these reforms.

Accountable Care Organizations

Section 3022 of the ACA created a government program to fund accountable care organizations (ACOs). ACOs are coordinated networks of physicians, hospitals, and other providers that strive to improve the provision of high-value primary care to a large group of Medicare patients. According to the law, ACOs are held responsible for the cost and quality of care for at least 5,000 Medicare patients. Since enactment of the ACA, Medicare has created several different types of ACOs to provide programs more carefully tailored to the financial, patient, practice, and other characteristics of the different medical organizations in the country (see Table 2.2, page 216).

In 2016, the ACOs were required to assess their performance against 34 quality measures such as screening for and treating high blood pressure and screening for depression. As an incentive, ACOs receive payments if they achieve quality targets and keep costs below a pre-established overall budget based on their patient population.

To date, there are more than 400 Medicare ACOs covering over 8 million Medicare beneficiaries. There are also approximately 700 ACOs that provide care to patients covered by private insurance companies. In general, ACOs have improved the quality of patient care, but their financial performance has been mixed. Importantly, the longer an ACO operates, the more likely it is to realize cost savings.

Whatever their ultimate impact, the inclusion of the ACO model in the ACA constitutes one step in the healthcare system's transition away from the fee-for-service model to one in which payment is tied to improving quality and controlling costs.

Center for Medicare and Medicaid Innovation (CMMI)

The authors of the ACA could not have anticipated all the potential types of payment and delivery system reforms that might reliably improve the quality of care and control costs. Therefore, Congress wisely institutionalized innovation by creating a unit within the Center for Medicare and Medicaid Services (CMS) that had the authority and resources to test out new models of payment and delivery of care: the Center for Medicare and Medicaid Innovation (CMMI). As section 3021 of the ACA stated, the "purpose of the CMMI is to test innovative payment and service delivery models to reduce program expenditures . . . while preserving or enhancing the quality of care furnished to individuals." CMMI was given $10 billion for this mission.

The creation of CMMI and its considerable resources was a strong signal that the federal government was serious about finding evidence-based alternatives to fee-for-service reimbursement that were capable of improving the value of Medicare. Its projects have offered different payment frameworks to help physicians and other medical organizations launch initiatives to improve quality and lower costs.

It is highly unusual for Congress to grant agencies the authority to make decisions that would otherwise require legislation. Usually this is only done when the decisions are important and the right policy answer faces substantial political challenges. In section 3021 of the ACA Congress gave the secretary of Health and Human Services (HHS) the authority to implement as a permanent policy change throughout Medicare and Medicaid any project conducted by the CMMI without having to ask Congress to pass a law. To implement such a change throughout the system, the Department of HHS Office of the Actuary must review the project's independent evaluation and certify that the payment or other program change, when widely implemented, would produce 1 of 3 results: (1) improve quality without increasing Medicare or Medicaid costs, (2) keep quality stable while saving money, or (3) both improve quality and save money.

This authority is both underappreciated and tremendously important. It helps to convince physicians, hospitals, and other providers that, if they succeed, CMMI's demonstration and pilot projects are likely to become permanent government policies. In short, if an ACO demonstration project or a bundled payment project generates cost savings, then it will be institutionalized. This provision reduces the risk for providers when they invest in transformation.

To date, the HHS secretary has invoked this 3021 authority only once to institute a diabetes prevention program (DPP) to begin payment in 2018. It is unclear how the Trump administration views both CMMI and this policy. Dr. Price has been vocal about his hostility to CMMI, but it is unclear that this aversion is shared by others who seem more focused on affordability and achieving high-value care. If CMMI stays under the Trump administration and the authority to implement demonstration projects nationally is used, physicians and hospitals will be further convinced that payment and delivery system change are not just rhetorical but real.

Hospital Readmission Policy

For years nearly 20% of Medicare patients discharged from hospitals were re-admitted within 30 days. This was true both at community hospitals and even at some of the country's most prestigious hospitals. Data suggested that this rate could be brought down if the care transitions were better managed and if the patient's primary care physician saw the patient within a few days of hospital discharge. And yet there remained woefully little coordination between hospitals and physicians at discharge. Hospitals would frequently discharge patients without even informing the primary care physician. Sometimes the primary care physician was informed but failed to make a timely follow-up appointment. Even when an appointment was made for a few days after discharge, the patient would often fail to show up. So for years and years the readmission rate did not decline.

The ACA tried to change these habits by financially penalizing hospitals that had high readmission rates. Initially, the penalty applied to readmissions after hospitalizations for acute health attacks, heart failure, or pneumonia. It was later expanded to include hospitalizations for hip or knee replacement surgery and emphysema, but still excluded planned readmissions, such as for cardiac surgery after admission for chest pain and a catheterization. The law escalated the penalty from 1%

of a hospital's payment from Medicare to 3% in 2015 and beyond. Given that hospital margins currently average 2.2%, this is serious financial punishment.

This policy has already had a beneficial impact on quality of care. An evaluation published in the *New England Journal of Medicine* in 2016 revealed a drop in total readmissions for acute heart attacks, heart failure, and pneumonia from 21.5% in 2007 to 17.8% in 2015. In addition, readmissions for all other conditions also dropped during this time. This trend was not just a continuation of the drop that began before the ACA; as the authors point out, "readmission rates began to fall faster in April 2010 after passage of the ACA than before." Unfortunately, the rate of decline did slow down after 2012, which suggests that we may be seeing a return to business as usual. Nonetheless, this policy has helped steer hospitals toward ensuring that patient transitions out of the hospital are more coordinated and that poor-quality, expensive care is reduced.

Hospital-Acquired Conditions

The Centers for Disease Control (CDC) estimates that 5% of patients become infected while in the hospital and that as many as 23,000 people die each year from hospital-acquired infections. This represents not only poor quality but also expensive care. For instance, developing pneumonia while on the ventilator adds over $20,000 to an average hospital bill. Infections are just one type of preventable injury that hospitalized patients experience. It was estimated that in 2010 "adult patients [in the United States] experienced roughly 4.8 million hospital-acquired conditions [over] 32.8 million hospital discharges." This is obviously a huge problem. Yet because hospitals were often paid for these infections and other complications, there was no real financial incentive driving them to address the situation.

To get hospitals to take this quality problem seriously, section 3008 of the ACA financially penalized hospitals in the worst-performing quartile by reducing their total Medicare payment by 1% and publicly reporting the poor results on the government's Hospital Compare website. In addition to infections, hospitals are assessed on pressure ulcers, falls, medication errors, and other preventable complications. Similar to the readmission policy, this penalty is a change in the law and policy rather than a demonstration project, that is, a permanent change.

The hospital-acquired condition policy went into effect on October 1, 2014. In 2015, of the 3,308 hospitals affected by this policy, 758 were penalized. Just over half are repeat offenders. Interestingly, some of the nation's best-known hospitals—Stanford, Denver Health Medical Center, and 2 hospitals affiliated with the Mayo Clinic—were among those penalized.

This policy uses payment penalties to focus hospitals' attention on improving the quality of care they deliver and, in particular, reducing costly and preventable injuries to patients. It is another step the ACA took to link payment to quality rather than to just the number of patients a hospital admits.

SINCE ITS PASSAGE in 2010 the ACA has done much to create a health policy foundation upon which the transformation of the delivery of healthcare can be built. The ACA is only the beginning. Subsequent policy changes have reinforced and magnified this change.

BUNDLED PAYMENTS FUEL TRANSFORMATION FOR SPECIALISTS

If fee-for-service is like ordering a dinner a la carte, a bundled payment is like getting a *prix fixe* dinner. A bundled payment is a single prespecified payment for a specific episode of care. It includes all payments to the physicians, the hospital, and sometimes for post-hospital care and other services. For instance, a bundled payment for hip replacement surgery might cover the cost of the presurgical evaluation, the surgeon, the anesthesiologist, the artificial hip implant, the hospital operating suite, the hospital room and board, intensive care unit (ICU) stays (if any), laboratory tests, and any other hospital costs such as blood transfusion(s), post-hospital rehabilitative services, and the costs associated with complications such as surgical-site infections.

Two main ideas underlie bundled payments. First, by receiving only 1 bundled payment, physicians and hospitals must coordinate care and reduce the unit costs to keep their overall costs below the fixed amount. Second, by being held financially responsible for complications, physicians and hospitals are encouraged to both standardize care and measure, report, and improve quality.

Before the ACA, experiments had demonstrated the potential for bundled payments to increase quality and lower costs. For instance, in January 2009 the Center for Medicare and Medicaid Services (CMS), the federal government agency that oversees Medicare, launched a bundled-payment initiative called the Acute Care Episode (ACE). It was a demonstration project that covered 37 cardiac and orthopedic procedures, such as bypass surgery, cardiac stents, pacemakers, and hip replacements, in 11 hospitals. The ACE demonstration project saved an average of $319 per person across 12,501 cases.

While working in the White House in 2009, I advocated for adding a provision to the ACA that would require CMS to implement at least 5 bundles. Unfortunately CMS opposed a legislative mandate for bundled payments, arguing that few physicians and hospitals were sufficiently aligned to accept this new form of payment.

I lost. Nothing in the ACA required expanding bundled payments to become a regular part of Medicare reimbursement. Over the last few years, however, CMMI has announced 4 major bundled-payment initiatives (see Table 2.3, page 217).

In July 2015, CMS created the Comprehensive Care for Joint Replacement Model (CJR), a bundled-payment initiative that covers hip and knee replacement surgery. CJR constitutes a major breakthrough in 3 respects. First, the episode payment covers inpatient hospital services, physician fees, and 90 days of care after the hospital discharge. This incentivizes high quality care, as the hospital is financially responsible for any complications, such as surgical-site infections, emergency room visits, and readmissions within 90 days. Second, CJR encourages reforming care following a hospitalization—so-called post-acute care—a field known to have wide and costly variation in care not justified by quality improvements. Third, CJR was the first mandatory demonstration project. It required nearly 800 hospitals to take part in the bundled-payment demonstration. This explicitly communicated to all hospitals and physicians, including specialists and surgeons, that payment really was changing and that they had to focus on transforming care. For this high-volume and highly profitable set of procedures, transformation of care was no longer optional.

Although the CJR model is a breakthrough, it still has 3 important limitations. One is that it pays hospitals rather than anyone who can provide the surgical and post-acute services. This gives more financial bargaining power to hospitals. Second, CJR does not permit surgical procedures in lower-cost ambulatory surgical centers, which are increasingly used for joint replacements. Finally, many people are concerned that bundles, reducing costs per unit of service, create a financial incentive to increase the number of episodes of care.

A second bundled-payment effort is the Oncology Care Model (OCM). Whereas CJR focuses on a high-cost surgical specialty, OCM applies bundled payments to a high-cost medical specialty, cancer care. OCM begins payment at the initiation of an episode of chemotherapy and covers 6 subsequent months of care. Participating practices must deliver more patient-focused care. This includes having a clinician—physician or nurse practitioner—available 24/7, with real-time access to the patients' records, developing a 13-point care plan with specific goals of treatment—for instance, whether the intent is to cure the cancer or to be palliative—and advanced care planning. To ensure high-quality care, the practices must also guarantee that their chemotherapy is consistent with national guidelines, such as the National Comprehensive Cancer Network's preferred chemotherapy regimens.

OCM offers several advantages. First, it is aimed at a high-cost medical specialty thereby signaling the government's interest in having all physicians, not just primary physicians, embrace transformation. Second, in OCM, oncologists receive a bonus to reduce a patient's total cost of care. Thus, they have a financial motive to develop cost-effective ways to care for patients, not just to choose lower-cost chemotherapy regimens. Oncologists may change how they care for chemotherapy side effects and choose radiation oncologists who offer lower-cost but still clinically effective radiation services. Third, CMS partnered with 16 commercial payers to aggregate more payments and increase the financial incentives for oncologists to transform their practices. In total, 190 oncology practices, comprising over 1,000 oncologists, enrolled in OCM. This is more than 10% of oncologists in the United States.

Most recently, in August 2016, CMS announced that it would create a mandatory bundled-payment model for 2 cardiac interventions: coronary artery bypass graft surgery (CABG) and acute myocardial infarction (AMI). This bundled payment has the advantage of focusing on both a high-cost surgical procedure and highly paid medical specialists.

MACRA INSTITUTIONALIZES TRANSFORMATION

While the ACA consumed most of the attention on healthcare policy, it was not the only major piece of health care legislation President Obama signed. On April 16, 2015, Congress passed another major law that received much less fanfare but overwhelming bipartisan support. The Medicare Access and CHIP Reauthorization Act garnered 92 votes in the US Senate and repealed the dysfunctional Sustainable Growth Rate (SGR) formula that had determined how much Medicare's payment to physicians would change from year to year. In its place MACRA provided for future increases in physician fees, but did so in a way—albeit complex—that highly incentivizes transforming the delivery of care to be of higher quality and lower cost.

From 2016 to 2019 physician payments will increase by 0.5% annually, with no link to any requirement that physicians improve care or reduce costs. Many experts have objected to this pay increase without a quid pro quo from physicians. MACRA then established a complex payment mechanism in which future increases in payment to physicians are linked to improving quality and more prudent resource utilization.

The default track is the Merit-based Incentive Payment System (MIPS). It applies to all physicians who stay in a traditional fee-for-service model. MACRA streamlines Medicare's quality and value programs into one MIPS score. Instead of Medicare's multiple small bonus-payment programs, such as the Physician Quality Reporting Program, there is now only one program, MIPS.

MIPS gives each physician one score based on their performance across 4 domains: quality, cost, use of electronic records, and clinical practice improvement activities. How these different domains are weighted in the one MIPS score will change over time, with increasing emphasis in the later years on resource utilization. Based on their MIPS score, physicians will receive either a bonus or cut in their Medicare payments. For instance, a high-performing physician will see a maximum of a 4% increase in Medicare payments in 2019. By 2022 the maximum percentage of change in Medicare payments will increase to 9%. Importantly, the MIPS changes to physician payments are supposed to be budget neutral, meaning the bonuses to high-performing physicians must be matched by the cuts to poorly performing physicians.

The other track is the Alternative Payment Model (APM), which includes those physicians who are accepting risk-based payments, such as primary care physicians participating in Next Generation ACOs or a specialist in one of the bundled-payment models, like CJR. To qualify for the APM track, physicians cannot simply share in savings; they must have some downside risk—that is, they must be financially responsible for paying back any costs that exceed the target price or capitated payment. Physicians must also use electronic health records and have their payment tied to quality metrics.

MACRA arranged the incentives to encourage physicians to participate in the APM track. Between 2019 and 2024 payments to physicians in the APM track will have a 5% annual bonus. For example, the fee-for-service payment for an orthopedic surgeon doing hip replacements in the CJR bundled-payment program will increase by 5% each year for 5 years. That is a huge increase and a massive incentive. Importantly, MACRA does not change the other bonus payments in the APM, thereby leaving the alternative payment arrangements in place to reward orthopedic surgeons for improving quality and saving costs.

The MACRA program is an explicit attempt to do 2 things. First, it closely links Medicare payment to quality and value. More importantly, it encourages physicians to move to alternative payment models in which they are at financial risk for spending too much and evaluated for the quality of their care. This policy preference is manifest in the 5% annual bonuses attached to the fee schedule from 2019 to 2024 for physicians opting for alternative payment models.

MACRA is separate from the Affordable Care Act. It was a uniquely bipartisan piece of legislation, and Tom Price, the new secretary of

Health and Human Services, was one of its champions. Even if the Republicans repeal parts of the ACA, MACRA will still exist. More importantly, the way MACRA works also reinforces the use of ACOs and bundled payments. This combination of bipartisan support and use of ACA payment changes means the incentive for medical organizations to transform their care will persist no matter what happens to the ACA. In addition, because one of the tracks entails alternative payment models being pioneered by CMMI under the authority of the ACA, it seems likely that the payment reform initiated by CMMI will continue. Whatever is done in terms of repeal and replace, the policy elements that serve as the foundation for transformation of the delivery of care will continue.

THE CHANGE IN LANGUAGE AND MINDSET: WHAT DOES IT MEAN?

Following the enactment of the ACA many physicians and hospital executives complained that they felt like they were in "2 boats" being pulled in opposite directions. They were largely paid fee-for-service, which incentivized them to do higher volumes of high-margin medical services, while simultaneously being encouraged to transform their practices to deliver high-value care. Many argued this was untenable. If they really did transform their processes of care, not only would it require significant investments, but they would also sacrifice revenue because their Medicare and commercial insurance reimbursement schemes heavily relied on the fee-for-service model. Until a substantial portion of their financial incentives changed to be risk based, they could not wholeheartedly transform their care.

The summer of 2016 represented a major turning point in this debate. MACRA had been passed, financially incentivizing all physicians to begin to transform their care by 2019. Then, a few months later, CMS announced the mandatory cardiac bundled-payment initiative for CABGs and AMIs. After these 2 events, something was different. As the Advisory Board, a consulting company, put it, a "shockwave hit the world of cardiovascular services." Many other experts said that the initiative finally marked the long-awaited "tipping point in the movement from fee-for-service to alternative payment models."

In short, in 2016 payment change was finally moving beyond the experimental phase. It was real. It was no longer a matter of *if* the system would change; the change was happening, and with the passage of MACRA, it moved beyond the point of no return. Indeed, consultants were arguing that physicians and administrators had to change their mindsets. Payment change could now be relied on by physicians and hospital administrators when designing strategic plans and investment priorities. There was no question that providers "now need to develop the data analysis infrastructure, cost management discipline, and care coordination capabilities" for a new type of care.

One noticeable result has been that everyone in healthcare—whether a physician, a hospital administrator, a nurse, a payer, a device or drug manufacturer, or even a medical equipment supplier—has begun speaking a new language. They all are now comfortable including in their standard pitches, slide decks, or talking points the vocabulary of transformation: the "triple aim," "value-based care" and "value-based payment models," "capitation," "population health," and "patient-centric care." Since mid-2016, these phrases have become the standard language of healthcare.

Comfort with these words and concepts is important. But what do they really mean?

Of course, we can give their formal definitions (see Table 2.4, page 219), but the real question is: What does the new jargon mean at the ground level? What does it really take for a physician's practice or a multispecialty group to be "patient-centric"? What does a physician practice need to actually do that it was not doing before to deliver "value-based" care? What is needed to deliver "population health"? What management and financial policies need to be in place to transform care? The next chapter aims to answer this last question before we consider the 12 transformational practices of highly effective medical organizations.

Chapter 3

SIX ESSENTIAL ELEMENTS
OF TRANSFORMATION

ASK ANYONE in healthcare what it takes to transform a health-care delivery organization, and they will probably list 3 neces-sary ingredients: leadership, culture, and data. Incorrect. These elements are important and maybe even necessary, but they alone are not sufficient to catalyze real transformation of a physician practice or health system. Indeed, I have found that there are actually 6 *essential* elements for transformation (see Table 3.1, page 220).

Some are necessary for transformation. For example, it is hard to see how any organization could transform without leadership and at least some data. It is likewise rare—though not impossible—for an incum-bent healthcare organization to transform without an existential crisis. But not all 6 elements are strictly necessary. While almost all organiza-tions that have transformed assume substantial or total financial risk for the health of their patients, a few have been able to transform and still operate largely under a fee-for-service payment system, primarily as a result of careful contract negotiations. Some organizations have not even significantly changed how they pay physicians, maintaining pay formulae that insulate physicians from financial risk. Instead, these organizations have relied on other ways of engaging their physicians in the transformation process.

Different organizations have emphasized and relied more on certain elements. For instance, at WESTMED, a 350-physician multispecialty group practice in Westchester, New York, governance—or what might be called "physician engagement"—is heavily emphasized. At Dean Clinic, headquartered in Madison, Wisconsin, physician-management alignment is more heavily emphasized. So for different organizations, different elements play key roles in their transformations.

The 6 essential elements of transformation can be divided into 2 groups, largely based on timing—that is, whether an element is initiated and occurs *before* the transformation process or arises *during* the transformation process itself. A catalyzing crisis and leadership are key to initiating the process of transformation, whereas physician-management alignment and physician compensation are the type of elements that get crafted—and refined—as transformation proceeds.

A CATALYZING CRISIS

Newton's First Law of Motion states that bodies at rest will stay at rest unless acted on by an outside force. In behavioral economics, this is labeled "inertia" or "status quo bias." Inertia is as relevant to human beings as it is to inanimate objects. We find permanent change difficult to achieve. We all know this to be true from our many failed New Year's resolutions. We initiate change only at special moments and only occasionally follow through to make them permanent habits. Only a crisis—a new medical event or diagnosis, for example—is likely to lead to a serious lifestyle change. A crisis allows us to comprehend that following the old way is more dangerous or costly than radically changing and thus gives us the motivation to sustain change.

Therefore, almost no existing physician practice or health system—an incumbent—will transform how it delivers care to patients unless forced to change. A multi-billion-dollar hospital system that is making a 5% or 7% profit (or "margin" in the case of nonprofit hospitals) and, based on its payer contract, projects similar profits into the near-term future is not inclined to transform itself. Life is too good. Similarly, a physician practice in which physicians make a comfortable salary and have reasonable working conditions is not eager to change how it provides care nor to reconfigure its processes of care. Such transformations would take work, and why expend that kind of energy and resources unless absolutely necessary?

Almost no one changes when things are going well. Why would they? They must, therefore, be *compelled* to change. As John Kotter, one of the world's leading experts on change, said,

> With good business results . . . convincing people of the need for change is much harder . . . [I]n the words of one former CEO of a large European company, [the only way to change] 'is to make the *status quo* seem more dangerous than launching into the unknown.' . . . When the urgency rate is not pumped up enough, the transformation process cannot succeed.

The kind of force typically necessary to induce a practice or health system to completely transform how it operates is a "near-death," existential experience. Things must be going so badly that the very existence of the practice or organization is called into question.

This sense of crisis characterized Dean Clinic's experience. Dean Health Plan—the insurance arm of the organization—was created in the early 1980s as a consequence of action by the Wisconsin state legislature. To break the stranglehold of the Blue Cross Blue Shield plan, the state mandated that state workers be offered a health maintenance organization (HMO) option. About 8 or 9 practices around the state began offering HMOs, including 3 in the state capital, Madison. Thus, the Dean Health Plan owned by the physicians at the Dean Clinic—the healthcare delivery arm—was born. At first, only people already receiving their care from Dean Clinic enrolled in the health plan; total enrollment in the insurance product was just under 20,000 members. As the years passed, enrollment steadily increased without any big changes. As one Dean executive said, "For the first 5 or 10 years, our role was purely patient aggregation."

Then, between 2004 to 2005, the crisis hit. Dean Health System experienced "2 underperforming years" during which it recorded significant losses. The financial problems exposed a dysfunctional governance structure. At the time there were 2 distinct boards, one for the Dean Health System and one for the Dean Clinic. The corporate board itself was a bit dysfunctional, as it lacked any board committees. One Dean executive remembers the management disarray:

Just to tell you how hosed up it was, we had a doctor board and a health system board. The CEO reported to the DHS [Dean Health System] board, and the chief administrative officer reported to the physician practice board. It was totally bizarre. The leadership team lacked clear lines of accountability. For instance, the chief administrative officer did not report to the CEO in the dual governance structure. And while the senior managers were talented people, they did not get along. They were talented individuals that were not a team with a clear focus and clear performance metrics.

There was widespread cynicism because many people perceived that decisions were "driven by individuals and shareholders [physicians] as opposed to what might be for the collective benefit of Dean Clinic." As Dean Clinic began losing money, it became clear that poor management and lack of a cohesive management team was at least partially to blame.

To rescue the situation, Dean realized that everything had to change. The 2 boards were merged into one, and the roles of Board chair and CEO were separated. The leadership team was also replaced: "The CEO left, our chief medical officer left . . . 4 of the top 5 positions, all but the chief financial officer, left." The Board and new senior management team developed a new 5-year strategic plan focused on transforming the organization. This management team describes how the transition was rolled out:

It felt like you were jumping off this cliff together. We just had to change, and change pretty drastically. We weren't really sure where we were headed. It's not like, "Oh, I know that if I do this, then something good will happen." You just knew if you didn't change, there was not going to be Dean anymore. We knew we were working toward the right thing.

What *exactly* was "the right thing" to work toward? The financial losses made clear that Dean had to focus on a system-wide effort to improve its cost structure while still maintaining its high quality. In short, Dean realized that they had to emphasize high-value care:

In 2006, when we sort of started on this journey, we did a strategic plan with 5 task forces. We really looked at what we call the value model. We always look at 5 objectives: the clinical quality, the appropriate cost, and then we look at the service aspect as well as the internal satisfaction of our employees and staff. Those are the prisms that we have used through the last 10 years.

Today Dean is among the nation's highest-ranked health-maintenance organizations. It is now a 5-star Medicare Advantage plan—the highest ranking, shared with only 12 other plans nationwide. Additionally, J.D. Power has ranked Dean highest among health plans in the Minnesota-Wisconsin region for the second year in a row. This is even more impressive given the fact that Dean has the lowest-cost silver plan on the Wisconsin health insurance exchange. All in all, Dean has undergone a pretty successful transformation in response to its crisis.

Like Dean, Kaiser Permanente Mid-Atlantic also had a near-death experience. By 2008, Kaiser Permanente Mid-Atlantic Medical Group was struggling so much that it had the Northern California Kaiser Permanente Medical Group take over. In essence, "the Mid-Atlantic Medical Group leadership did a courageous thing. They put themselves out of a job and sought help because they were failing miserably." How did it come to this?

Since 1980, Kaiser had had a presence in the Washington, DC–Maryland-Virginia area, but it never seemed to "take" the same way that the plan did in California and Oregon (see Chapter 8). By 2008, years of management missteps, a lack of a strategic vision, and chronic underinvestment all came together to create what people at Kaiser still refer to as "The Crisis":

> Membership was dropping and had been steadily dropping year after year for about 10 years. Kaiser Permanente Mid-Atlantic had a poor reputation in the market. The region was eking out its margin targets, very low-margin targets, but it was doing so by very poor internal investments. There was no investment in facilities and people. For instance, there were completely inadequate numbers of primary care physicians.

The medical group management structure was disorganized and dys-functional. Before the transformation, you could be an allergist in Virginia and report to somebody in Baltimore, who never saw you, never met with you, and there's a little bit of the "out of sight, out of mind." You did not know the people that you were being led by. You did not know the people that you were leading.

Unless something drastic changed, Kaiser Permanente Mid-Atlantic was going to go out of business. In 2008, Dr. Bernadette Loftus, a head and neck surgeon, was dispatched by the Kaiser Permanente Medical Group in northern California to turn around the region. Loftus insti-tuted a wide variety of changes, prioritized according to how immedi-ately necessary they were. One set of changes focused on hiring more primary care physicians to decrease the panel size to about 1,950 pa-tients per internist or family physician. This allowed patients to book appointments whenever they wanted and gave physicians sufficient time to treat patients. The new team also focused on improving spe-cialty care. As Loftus explained,

> Patients in this region have a very high bar for access to specialists. They want to see a specialist when they think they need to see a specialist. And it doesn't really matter frankly whether it's technically medically necessary or not. So you might as well take care of the problem, soothe the psyche of the worried well upfront rather than generate anger by bouncing them around the system trying to get in.

Next the Loftus team shifted their attention to improving performance measurement and, through such changes, also improving the quality of care.

Today Kaiser Permanente Mid-Atlantic is a 5-star Medicare Advantage plan that ranks first in the nation for a laundry list of NCQA quality met-rics—from over 90% of members with blood pressure control to over 90% of age-appropriate women receiving breast cancer screening. Ac-cording to J.D. Power, Kaiser Permanente Mid-Atlantic has also received the highest ranking in overall member satisfaction among commercial health plans in mid-Atlantic states. The organization is yet another ex-ample of how a crisis is necessary to facilitate successful transformation.

At WESTMED, a medical group in Westchester County, New York, the "crisis" was the proliferation of managed-care organizations in the early 1990s combined with the threat of "Hillary Care"—the Clinton healthcare reform proposal. As Simeon Schwartz, the CEO of WESTMED, explains,

> In the early 1990s, we thought the country was going to move to a complete value-based system. . . . It was obvious to me that with the rapid expansion of managed care and the new health reforms being proposed by the Clinton administration, some form of capitation was imminent. The only way to function would be to focus on reducing costs and improving quality because physicians would be held accountable for the total cost of care.

Then the Clinton health reform proposal failed. Managed care induced a backlash. While many groups were left scrambling, WESTMED had already set itself out on a path of transformation. As Schwartz describes it, "We got dressed up for the prom and we were stood up for 20 years. You can imagine what my corsage looked like all those years later." Although WESTMED may have overanticipated their "crisis," their early changes ultimately worked wonders.

Since the ACA's initiation of policy changes and subsequent governmental actions, new players have entered the field offering better primary healthcare. These newcomers include groups like Iora Health, VillageMD, and Aledade. As new entrants, they are responding not to an internal crisis but rather to a crisis in the larger healthcare environment—the crisis of underperformance and unaffordability of healthcare. These new companies have tried to offer an alternative in a stagnant healthcare environment plagued by minimal innovation and great dissatisfaction with the quality, cost, and patient experience of care.

LEADERSHIP

Leadership is another absolutely necessary element for transformation. Even in the face of a crisis, the steps needed for transformation do not happen spontaneously. Without a leader, it is hard to see how a practice or health system could organically transform. Someone has to be pushing the change forward and deciding on the direction of the change. Someone has to wake up every day, figuring out what is needed to make that change happen, and communicating the way forward. In this sense, leadership is about high-level strategic vision and direction and is distinct from management, which keeps the ship afloat. In Kotter's words,

> Management's mandate is to minimize risk and keep the current system operating. Change, by definition, requires creating a new system, which in turn always demands leadership.

Leadership is therefore highly important—but that is different from saying that leadership can transform an organization alone. Leadership, although necessary, is not sufficient—there are, as we know, these other essential elements. Nevertheless, leadership does seem to be one of those necessary foundational elements of transformation. Each successful practice or health system had a leader or leaders who spearheaded the change that ultimately transformed the organizations.

The leaders profiled in this book embody 2 key attributes, characteristics that experts have identified as critical to successfully guiding an organization: analytical skills and emotional intelligence.

Leaders equipped with analytic skills are able to imagine and communicate a compelling, long-term, strategic vision for their practice or health system. They see where the American healthcare system is headed and what their practice or health system must do to succeed in that future. In addition, they can prioritize effectively. They do not try to do everything at once. They know what must be done to initially push transformation and what should be left to the next tier of transformation and then the next. As Loftus emphasized, transforming Kaiser Permanente Mid-Atlantic required prioritization of what to fix first:

> This was a failing region in 2008. . . . I think there was a failure of leadership. You know, in a way, leaders can fail. There was also what I would say was a lack of the basic blocking and tackling that you have to do to run a healthcare delivery system. So, in this order, we worked on analytics, leadership restructure, primary-care hiring, specialty access, and only then did we go for quality.

Loftus focused on the most pressing problems—primary care delivery, leadership, and data analytics—before moving on to quality and hospital contracts. Since implementing these changes, Kaiser Permanente Mid-Atlantic has begun to focus on understanding how it is doing in achieving its objectives. It now has statistics and cases at its fingertips that allow it to know where the organization is succeeding in achieving its goals and where it is falling short and needs to do better.

The second key attribute of good leaders is emotional intelligence skills (EQ). As one of the leadership experts explained,

> Analytics and technical skills do matter, but mainly as "threshold capabilities"—that is, they are the entry-level requirements for executive positions. But . . . emotional intelligence is the sine qua non of leadership. Without it, a person can have the best training in the world; an incisive, analytical mind; and an endless supply of smart ideas, but he still won't make a great leader.

All of the leaders mentioned in this book have great EQ, which allows them to gather and effectively run a management team and execute their objectives.

Emotional intelligence is one of those capacious phrases that encompass many things, perhaps erroneously so. It is very important to differentiate EQ from analytic skills and IQ, which are both heavily—and maybe too heavily—emphasized in healthcare. For this book's leaders EQ is characterized by 3 critical elements. One is motivation. These leaders want their organizations to excel. They realize that they personally succeed only when their organization succeeds. As Jim Collins, business consultant and author of *From Good to Great*, a book about what makes great companies and organizations, puts it when characterizing leaders of great companies, "They are incredibly ambitious—but their ambition is first and foremost for the institution, not themselves." The actions of these leaders are not all about the "I." They all, of course, have their own egos, but they see their success as a reflection of the success of their organization. Individual success is not what drives the leaders of medical organizations toward transformation; instead, they want to build something bigger than themselves, something that could both deliver high-value care to patients and satisfy employees by offering them meaningful work. This desire is not something these leaders only repeat in their stock speeches; it runs deep. For instance, when asked about what kind of role his leadership played in making WESTMED successful, Schwartz continually deflected the opportunity to crow, instead emphasizing governance, rather than leadership, as the root of his organization's success. Leaders like Simeon are motivated to get positive results and then to show such results to the world. They do not want only moral victories but also actual, meaningful, measurable change that others can grasp and appreciate.

All of the leaders mentioned in this book love a challenge and are motivated by challenges to excel. They are not ruffled by failure. These leaders are both sure of their visions and recognize that realizing these goals may not be a straight shot. They do not expect everything to always succeed. These leaders expect setbacks and understand the need for constant refinement and revision of their implementations. They don't expect their algorithms to always be right and are always willing to update them. Many of these leaders have also changed how their physicians are paid, though this transformation has often been bumpy and in need of frequent adjustments. Ultimately, the leaders in this book are both goal oriented *and* adaptable.

Leaders also must have empathy. In particular, successful leaders focus on understanding their patients' health, experiences, and feelings. Thus, they spend considerable effort trying to "get into the heads" of their patients in order to figure out how to make the system work for them.

No healthcare organization can succeed without its physicians. Therefore, the best leaders spend time trying to understand their physicians—what annoys them, what satisfies them, how to motivate them—and put that into practice.

Finally, leaders are natural team builders. They assemble driven colleagues into teams, bringing out the best in each colleague individually and the group as a whole. Leaders also encourage these teams to collaborate in pursuit of the organization's goals. They have the communication and social skills necessary to encourage group activities and are willing to fire those unable to commit to the organization's goals. Similarly, leaders hire with the team's benefit in mind. They want people who are both analytically skilled and able to work effectively within the organization as team players. Many of these leaders emphasize that they hire for empathy and EQ because "the rest can be taught."

Contrary to Tolstoy's claim in *Anna Karenina* that "happy families are all alike; every unhappy family is unhappy in its own way," the right leaders are not all the same. Indeed, the analytic and EQ skills that make a successful leader can come in many different packages. Some of the leaders I encountered, for example, are larger-than-life characters. Sheldon Zinberg of CareMore is a bubbly, Catskills-style comedian who can sometimes be deemed "provocative" in today's politically correct culture. One colleague even called Zinberg "the Wolf of Wall Street in healthcare." He comes up with scores of disruptive ideas, some of which he readily admits might seem wacky, but he displays curiosity and deep, unconventional thinking. One of his more recent ideas is "Neurodynamic Fitness Training." He believes special exercise programs can improve neurogenesis, neuroplasticity, and the secretion of neurotransmitters ultimately to improve cognitive skills. This idea has driven him to advocate that every senior at CareMore be enrolled in his specialized "neurodynamic" training regimen.

Simeon Schwartz of WESTMED is another larger-than-life leader. Schwarz is an engaging, high-energy speed-talker with a million ideas and a great sense of humor, often at his own expense. Other leaders are of the quieter, more analytic variety. John Sprandio, a mild-mannered practicing oncologist, is naturally trusted by fellow physicians and was even elected by a large group to lead them into the future. Others, like Bernadette Loftus and Allison Mooney of Dean Clinic, exude more collaborative mentalities and are openly admired by their colleagues for their calm leadership. But no matter how it is outwardly manifested, all exhibit the same combination of great analytic skills and emotional intelligence that has helped them realize the full potential of their organizations.

Does the leader have to be a physician? It helps, but it is not necessary. Historically, nonmedical personnel have had a hard time managing physicians. Throughout the 20th century, most physicians attempted to maintain their autonomy by organizing themselves into small independent practices rather than banding together inside larger, top-down medical groups. They seemed willing to listen only to one another, viewing outside managers as incapable of appreciating the trials of their extensive training, the experience of caring for seriously ill and dying patients, their well-honed judgment and dedication, and their "pure," nonmonetary motivations as physicians.

As "insiders," physician-leaders can more easily circumvent these suspicions. Because of their shared experience in the trenches of patient care, they are endowed with the credibility, as one such leader put it, "to communicate the 'why' behind what has to be done in a way that their fellow physicians can understand." Hence, it is true that most of the leaders in transformed organizations are physicians—like Sheldon Zinberg, Simeon Schwartz, John Sprandio, Bernadette Loftus, Chris Chen of ChenMed and Lee Sacks of Advocate in Chicago. But not all. Allison Mooney at Dean Clinic and Leeba Lessin at CareMore are 2 nonphysician leaders who are highly talented executives. (In the case of Mooney, physicians were part of the leadership team.) But what made them effective is that, despite their lack of medical background, they had the ability to empathize with, engage, and, thereby, win over physicians. Therefore, it appears that at least part of a nonphysician-leader's success lies in being able to understand physicians. The other part, as one leader put it, is "transparency, putting up metrics for all to see and performing against them." At Dean Clinic, for example, the physician deference to Mooney was.

CULTURE, GOVERNANCE, AND PHYSICIAN ENGAGEMENT

"Culture eats strategy for breakfast, lunch, and dinner," is a common management maxim. It is popular because it embodies an important truth. A positive and constructive culture willing to change is essential to success. Still, much like organizational strategy, culture is not immutable: it can change and evolve.

What is the culture of an organization? Culture is the ethos that characterizes the organization, the driving mission that all employees imbibe and use to guide the way they perform their jobs. Experts say that organizational culture is instantiated through 6 components: vision, values, practices, people, narrative, and place.

Each organization has a slightly different tone and uses slightly different expressions to capture its vision of transformed care. Although they might phrase it differently, medical organizations that have transformed the way they care for patients all have adopted certain key values as central to their organization: they excel at the quality of care, they have controlled and even lowered the total cost of care, they have improved the patient experience, and they have improved employee work satisfaction. These values animate everything these organizations do. They are not just oft-repeated phrases or abstract ideas; rather, they are real touchstones embedded in the organization's strategic goals and tactical decisions. They permeate every custom and procedure that guides the care experience, human resource policies, and other organizational practices. They are what employees fall back on when making judgments in ambiguous situations. Everyone knows them and can connect how they justify key decisions with the policies of the practice or organization.

Obviously to be effective these values must be authentic and not just phrases thrown around to promote an organization. Leaders in the organization must embody these values and help their employees believe in and affirm them. It is important that all employees—nurses, medical assistants, administrative staff, and others—adopt these values. Many successful organizations set aside a specific time at the start of each day or week for a team huddle on the most challenging, chronically ill patients or the high-cost, high-risk patients in order to communicate to employees the importance of providing high-value care. Similarly, empowering medical assistants to close care gaps and having nurse practitioners perform annual physical exams communicates the value of lowering the cost of care and improving the patient experience. Assessing employee performance on these tasks further emphasizes their fundamental importance.

It is most important for physicians to affirm and espouse their organization's core values. Physicians are the most crucial patient caregivers—they are the ones who write the orders for tests, treatments, office visits, and hospital admissions, the ones who ultimately define a patient's quality and total cost of care. If the physicians do not aspire to and work toward achieving the highest-possible quality of care and patient experience, transformation will not happen. Conversely, physicians who affirm the importance of higher-quality and low-er-cost care and are engaged in choosing their performance metrics and improving their performance will both explicitly and implicitly encourage their colleagues to follow their example. This is why, despite the considerable differences among the numerous value-oriented or-ganizations, virtually all emphasize physician governance and engage-ment. By doing so, these organizations induce physician buy-in to the goals of transformation and the necessary steps to achieve those goals. Schwartz describes how this mentality works at WESTMED:

> We ask our physicians how you want to manage this medical condition. We ask our physicians to come up with the criteria for evaluation and build a form. They come up with the consensus, and the problems with inconsistent management of clinical conditions go away.
>
> This is the bottom-up, self-governing model without authoritative management. It is built on the principles of both high quality and low costs, and it empowers doctors.
>
> By the way, it is one of the reasons our physicians are all happy.

THESE ORGANIZATIONS all have similar narratives surrounding their visions and missions. They generally acknowledge the presence of a cri-sis and how their response transformed the organization. Or, if they are a newer group, they talk about how they saw a gaping hole in the ex-isting healthcare system that was adversely affecting patients—the sys-tem's crisis—and understood how their company could fill that hole.

Finally, there is the value of place. Both the location and interior de-sign of buildings can help shape culture. This phenomenon is some-thing that health systems, with their maze-like collections of buildings and cookie-cutter offices, often overlook. Many transformed practices, however, have taken architecture and design seriously. For instance, while WESTMED's large polyclinics are housed in nondescript office buildings, the interior design was meticulously thought out to ensure a calm, attentive experience for WESTMED patients. As Dr. Schwartz, the CEO, explains,

> Here we are in the patient waiting area. We want you to have a Zen mo-
> ment. There are two things to notice. Number one, the changing dis-
> plays of nature on the large TV monitors scattered around. Number
> two, listen to the noise level. Absolutely quiet.

Likewise, when Dean Clinic was building a new clinic, they named
patients and staff to the design committee to ensure that their values
were incorporated into the building itself. For instance, patients said
they wanted a "one-stop-shop" feel to the clinic, so an eyeglass store
was included in the new office building. Similarly, physicians and nurse
practitioners were placed in adjoining offices with an opening between
them to facilitate teamwork. In the same way, CareMore also took steps
to embed its culture in the physical layout of its facilities by placing
its exercise studios, called Nifty after Fifty (pages 158–161, 220), immediately adjacent to the medical offices. Such co-location sends a powerful message about the organization's commitment to lifestyle interventions and prevention as part of its larger care plan and it implicitly
communicates—both to staff and to patients—that wellness promotion is an integral part of the organization's mission.

DATA

Like leadership, data is an absolutely necessary management element
for transformation. Indeed, one of the most important elements distin-
guishing the 1990s "managed care" era and today's healthcare reform
efforts is data. We now have a lot more worthwhile data that can inform change. These data can help organizations understand their practices, assess their performance against benchmarks, identify deficiencies, implement solutions, and, again, evaluate their impact.

It used to be that almost every practice or organization that tried to
transform suffered pushback with regards to the data they were using
to inform their proposed changes. Physicians were particularly adept
at raising a number of classic arguments. The traditional litany of objections usually began with the claim that "you don't have the data."
But when the data were produced, physicians then claimed that "the

data are out of date." When the data were proven to be up to date, the objection changed to "the data are garbage; they are inaccurate." Even when accuracy was established and data were risk adjusted, physicians *still* complained that "the data are inadequate. Claims data can't capture relevant clinical information, such as stage of cancer." The objections were, in short, endless.

It is true that there can always be more and better data. Current claims-based, risk-adjustment methodologies are far from optimal. And, yes, given the siloing of electronic records data, it *is* often difficult to merge and synthesize accurate clinical data. But we cannot reify "data" and allow the fact that it is always possible to identify data deficiencies to impede care transformation. We are now squarely passed the threshold; we have sufficient data to begin—and carry out for a significant time—the process of transformation. So long as we are willing to work with the data we have, we can also simultaneously improve the amount and quality of the data.

I will not further discuss data, IT systems, electronic health records (EHRs), interoperability, and the myriad other issues associated with getting better data for care transformation. Many other commentators are more proficient on these particular issues. What is important to emphasize here is that care transformation does require ready access to data—in particular, to 5 types of data. First, organizations must have access to claims data that are updated on a periodic, preferably monthly basis. It would be ideal to have utilization on a real-time basis, and many practices and organizations do have such data. But monthly claims data are sufficient for clinical care and assessments of quality of care and costs. Second, laboratory data are critical to clinical care. Such data should be available electronically on a real-time basis for providers using appropriate EHRs. Third, organizations need real-time access to imaging studies and reports. These data are electronic and should be available in real time. The important issue for clinical management is to have all imaging from all facilities available immediately after the tests are performed. This requires overcoming much of the interoperability problem. Fourth, real-time pharmacy data—knowing what drugs a patient is taking and whether they are refilling their prescriptions—are necessary to understand utilization, adherence, cost, and other aspects of care. Finally, organizations should collect data on admissions and discharges from hospitals, skilled nursing facilities, and other institutions. This is currently the weakest of the available data, as it is often either not shared at all, or shared in a lackadaisical manner that prevents timely action. Indeed, economic incentives drive many hospitals and other facilities not to share these data. Additionally, many EHRs are not yet interoperable, thereby preventing timely sharing of these data. Experts expect that over the next few years interoperability will become the norm, and these data will become readily available.

Organizations that have successfully transformed face the challenge of converting these data into useable sources for 2 different functions. One is to inform physicians, nurse practitioners, and other front-line providers in real time about the clinical status of their patients. It is important that providers know about recent ER visits, hospitalizations, and other medical interventions. It is also vital to know in real time about any new laboratory and imaging results. This information has to be in a format that is accessible for the clinician during a patient encounter. In the words of oncologist John Sprandio, clinicians must be "data users, not data miners." In short, given that physicians already have precious little face-to-face time with patients, they should not be expected to also occupy that time with searching around a patient's electronic chart for relevant data. Physicians need to have the laboratory, imaging, pharmacy, and other data readily at hand for immediate use during a visit to make informed clinical decisions.

The other critical function is performance measurement. This largely requires access to 3 types of data: claims and cost data on ER use, hospitalization rates, imaging rates, referral rates, and the like; data on pharmacy utilization, such as use of beta blockers, aspirin, lipid-lowering agents, ACE inhibitors, and other drugs prescribed after heart attacks; and some clinical data, such as a patient's HgA1c and blood pressure. Much of this is readily available to practices or can be obtained from EHR data. As we will see in Chapter 4, the key step is converting the data to show physicians how they are performing relative to both their peers and national norms, all in a manner that can positively influence their practices. Doing so is feasible, especially when it is acknowledged that accessing such data is not impossible.

We currently *do* have access to sufficient data for transformation. Lack of access to data still might be an excuse not to act, but it is no longer a real barrier to transformation.

PHYSICIAN-MANAGEMENT ALIGNMENT

One important element of transformation that is often ignored especially in larger group practices and health systems is the collaboration between managers and physicians. Although physicians may want a specific change, it is up to managers to actually facilitate the creation of the necessary infrastructure. Equipped with this infrastructure, physicians must then change their practices. For instance, if physicians no longer want to be responsible for ensuring that patients are getting their mammograms, and Pap smears and instead want the "system" to take over this function, the managers need to put an alternative process in place. Similarly, if physicians develop a standardized protocol for managing atrial fibrillation, then the managers need to ensure that resources are devoted to creating and deploying standard orders sets in both the EHR and the compliance program.

Dean Clinic effectively addressed this issue of physician-management alignment during its transformation journey. In 2005, before its crisis and transformation, Dean was a governance nightmare. There was no clear accountability and the emphasis was on production, seeing ever more patients.

One of Dean Clinic's more important management changes was the creation of "physician-administrator dyads." At every level of the organization there was an effort to "pair operations leadership and management with a physician partner . . . to work both sides of the equation, both the medical delivery and the operations side of it." The physician offers care providers a voice while simultaneously translating managers' needs back to the frontline physicians and other providers as well as working to secure physician buy-in. The administrator works to ensure that the necessary resources—financial, physical, information technology, and human—are secured and deployed for any initiative. Examples of dyads include the physician who heads the board's finance committee with the chief financial officer, and the chief medical officer with the chief operating officer. This management structure has been replicated throughout the Dean Health System. The regional medical director and the regional administrator are paired. In medical divisions, such as orthopedics and primary care, there are also physician-administrator pairs. At each clinical site, a physician site chief and a clinic manager are paired. In addition, the physician and administrator's performance metrics and compensation bonuses are aligned. Because both are formally and explicitly responsible for the same outcomes, this alignment reinforces their shared interests and encourages them to work together to achieve mutual goals.

Although Dean's dyad structure is not necessary for transformation, some physician-administrator performance and bonus alignment certainly makes the process progress more smoothly.

FINANCIAL INCENTIVES

For a long time, I thought it was impossible for a medical organization to transform while still being paid predominantly fee-for-service. But the real issue is not the payment type itself, but how the financial incentives are structured and whether they are transmitted not just to the medical organization but to physicians and other providers who are delivering the actual patient care.

Financial risk comes in different shapes and sizes. Capitation is obviously the purest form, but financial risk can take the form of bundled payments for specific treatments, or courses of treatment, or can even be thought of as being held responsible for the total cost of patient care, with financial penalties in place should a given budget be exceeded. Typically the capitated amount—or the portion of the savings of the total cost of care—that is shared with the physicians or health system is tied to both quality and performance metrics in order to reduce incentives to skimp either on care and patients' care experiences. Therefore, practices and health systems stand to make money by improving both the quality of care and patient experience while also controlling costs. Likewise, they will lose money if they continue to operate as though they are compensated in a fee-for-service manner, doing more tests and treatments, regardless of quality or appropriateness, in the hopes of running up the bill. The risk side of this equation—the threat of losing money if they spend too much—is particularly powerful and is thought by many to be indispensable to incentivizing transformation. The behavioral economics principle of loss aversion highlights that people value losses more than gains. Losses—or even threats of losses—are inherently more motivating. Thus, the threat of losing money is likely to act as a more powerful incentive for change than the promise of additional gains. This loss aversion is central to incentivizing the transformation of the delivery of care.

Most practices or health systems that have transformed themselves have financial risk arrangements. While they have a dual administrative structure, Kaiser Permanente and Group Health of Puget Sound (now part of the Kaiser family) are both fully integrated delivery systems and the organization directly links both the health insurer and the health provider. They both take in premiums and operate the health system. If their operations exceed the premiums, they will lose money. Similarly, at Dean Clinic about half of the patients are part of the Dean Health Plan, a traditional health-maintenance organization that takes their premium. Dean also offers insurance on the Wisconsin exchange and so is at financial risk for these patients. Meanwhile CareMore is a Medicare Advantage health plan. It, too, gets a fixed premium for delivering all medical services to its Medicare patients. ChenMed receives fixed-rate contracts from Medicare Advantage health plans, particularly Humana. Advocate Health Care cobrands a health insurance plan with the local Blue Cross Blue Shield plan on the Illinois insurance exchange. Because Advocate's payment is fixed by the premium, it stands to lose if costs exceed premiums. Advocate also has a substantial Medicare Advantage population for which they are at full financial risk. Donna Medical Clinic, part of the Rio Grande Valley ACO, and the Aledade practices are in the Medicare MSSP program and participate in a shared savings arrangement (see pages 214, 216, 219).

Despite the examples listed above, there *are* ways to transform care under certain fee-for-service systems. WESTMED, for example, mostly operates using fee-for-service contracts. Although most of Aledade's physician practices are participating in Medicare's ACO program, they also have fee-for-service contracts with commercial insurers. Similarly

VillageMD has fee-for-service contracts with commercial insurers. How can these primary care clinics and multispecialty groups transform themselves when paid on a fee-for-service basis, which we traditionally think of as only incentivizing doing more regardless of the quality of the outcomes and appropriateness of services?

These groups typically are in fee-for-service arrangements with a twist, although the twists do not generally include financial loses. For instance, it is possible to negotiate higher fee-for-service payments in exchange for lower overall costs or other metrics that are tied to cost. WESTMED, for example, has negotiated very high rates for prenatal and delivery services. They are able to charge such high rates because the rates are tied to low utilization of neonatal intensive care units for premature infants. WESTMED achieves this by having excellent prenatal care that lowers premature births and complications. Thus, quality is improved and total costs are low, even though the fee-for-service payment to WESTMED is high for obstetric care.

Similarly, Aledade has been able to organize their primary care physicians and negotiate with commercial insurers for a gainshare in certain areas. The primary care practices are paid fee-for-service, but if they lower total costs of care, then the insurers pay them a share of the savings. This payment arrangement does not put the practices at financial risk—they can only make more by saving money on the total cost of care. Nevertheless, the arrangement incentivizes transformation.

Financial risk that includes incentives to not just reduce costs but also improve quality and patient experience has proven to be the best way to incentivize transformation. But as some practices demonstrate, it is possible to incentivize transformation using fee-for-service payment, albeit a "modified" fee-for-service arrangement with gainsharing or financial bonuses to ensure lower costs.

One of the biggest challenges that transforming practices and health systems must confront is how to communicate financial risks at the organizational level down to front-line physicians and other clinicians. Organizations usually assume the financial risk—as health-maintenance organizations, through premiums or capitated contracts, or by being held responsible for total cost of care. The clinicians are often still paid on a fee-for-service basis. This again creates the "2 boat" problem, but this time it is inside the practices or health system. Here the system is bearing financial risk while its clinicians are financially incentivized to do more.

At this point in the evolution of the American healthcare system even the most experienced organizations undergoing transformation are still experimenting with how best to pay—and incentivize—their physicians and other clinicians. Most organizations are trying ad hoc policies that are frequently being modified without much rigorous evaluation. For instance, Dean Clinic initially added to its fee-for-service payments to physicians a compensation component based on patient satisfaction. Then it tried to shift off fee-for-service while maintaining productivity by tying payment to the primary care physicians to their panel sizes, namely the number of patients attributed to the physician, fee-for-service billings (RVUs), with quality and cost performance components. As one Dean manager explains,

> [We are experimenting with] incentives for primary care that are more on quality outcomes and using evidence-based pathways of care. . . . [We are also integrating] more and more team metrics . . . so as not to disincentivize people from hiring lower-cost care team members to assist in managing a population of patients.

At Dean, physician compensation is still a work in progress.

Advocate Health Care also emphasizes team care in its incentive program. The financial incentives for its primary care physicians are 70% based on individual performance and 30% based on the medical team performance. However, the Advocate leadership readily admits that though this divide seems about right, it was conjured out of thin air and has not been subject to evaluation of its actual impact. In addition, the financial incentive does not apply to nonphysician team members, such as nurse practitioners, medical assistants, pharmacists, and others. Whether or not dividing the incentive among the team would be helpful has not been evaluated.

CareMore, meanwhile, bases up to 60% of pay to its extensivists—hospitalists who also follow and care for the sickest, chronically ill patients once they are discharged from the hospital—on 2 factors: short hospital lengths of stay and low readmission rates. This is a large financial incentive. Importantly, it not only incentivizes rapid discharges to save money but also ensures that patients are not leaving too soon and have the right posthospital services when discharged to either a skilled nursing facility or back home. Once again, however, this payment calculation is empiric and not the result of careful evaluation.

As more practices and health systems transform their delivery of care, whether and how they apply financial risk to physicians and front-line clinical staff—and whether the incentive applies to quality alone or quality, cost, and patient experience—will remain an issue in need of additional inquiry. It is an area in the midst of experimentation and evolution, but hopefully over the next 5 to 10 years more evidence for better—if not optimal—practices will emerge.

OVER THE next 10 years many physician practices, multispecialty groups, and health systems will confront the decision of whether or not to transform. They will have the option of assuming financial risk for their patients, whether through bundled payments, capitation, or other arrangements. They will have to put some, if not all, of these 6 essential elements in place—a catalyzing crisis; leadership; culture, governance, and physician engagement; data; physician-management alignment; and financial incentives. Once these elements are in place, the practice or health system will then have to figure out what to do. What does it mean to transform the delivery of care to patients? What actual steps should the leader suggest to the organization? How can a practice improve quality for chronically ill patients while controlling costs? Given the large number of changes that could be made, which changes should be given top priority and which should occur further down the road?

The next 3 chapters examine 12 practices of transformation that span every facet of care—from scheduling and rooming patients in an office, to the standardization of practices and chronic care management, to behavioral health, palliative care, and lifestyle interventions. I have identified these specific practices after examining many different transformed healthcare organizations across the United States and determining what habits they consistently perform to deliver higher-quality, lower-cost care that also improves patient experience with healthcare. Throughout my visits, I discovered that the transformed organizations have adopted similar—though not necessarily identical—approaches. Together they offer a roadmap for change—namely, the strategic direction to follow, the specific practices to implement, and in roughly what order.

Chapter 4

THE TWELVE PRACTICES
OF TRANSFORMATION

Transforming the Physician Office Infrastructure

T HE ACA, subsequent payment reform demonstration projects, and the enactment of MACRA have laid the policy and financial foundations for transforming the US healthcare delivery system. Together these federal initiatives have changed the psychology of all those in healthcare. Providers and payers alike now acknowledge that the system is inextricably moving toward rewarding higher-quality and lower-cost care. While congressional Republicans and the new Administration have created some uncertainty about what additional legislation and regulations might alter the path going forward, the direction ultimately remains clear. It is obvious that the US healthcare system is not going back to its old fee-for-service way, unaccountable for quality and total cost of care. Successful medical organizations of the future will be the ones that can consistently deliver high-value care and prove it through their performance data.

In light of this future, many physician practices and health systems want to change. They want to avoid having to face that near-death experience so many transformed practices have had to endure. Hence, they have begun to put in place the management essentials, leadership team, data, physician engagement, and payment contracts necessary for higher-quality, lower-cost care. They are talking to their employees about achieving the triple aim and the need for more patient-centric, high-value, population-based care.

These organizations want to transform the way they deliver care, yet they are uncertain about how to actually do so. What are the first few steps they need to take to transform their care? How should they go about changing their care delivery in the most responsible way?

This chapter, and Chapters 5 and 6, are an answer to their questions. By studying numerous practices and systems, I have identified 12 transformational practices that medical organizations that want to change to patient-centric, high-value care should implement (see Table 4.1, page 222). They are listed in order of how patients interact with the healthcare system, from scheduling an appointment and registering at the office to receiving palliative care and lifestyle interventions. Because no organization can implement all 12 transformational practices at once, I have also delineated 3 tiers of transformation, a general sequence of when to implement each practice (pages 189–194). We begin with those practices that transformed the physician office infrastructure. Then in Chapter 5, move to how different providers—physicians, hospital, skilled nursing facilities, and others—interact to improve care. Finally, we look at how the traditional medical care model can be enhanced with behavioral health, palliative care, and other types of services in Chapter 6.

PRACTICE 1: SCHEDULING A PATIENT APPOINTMENT

I recently needed to see my primary care physician for a follow-up examination. My kidney function needs to be checked each year and had not been monitored since the previous spring. On April 4, I used an online email link built into my health system's EHR (electronic health record) to request a physician office visit. The next day, the scheduling person emailed me back, saying,

> I scheduled you to see Dr. Wilson on May 24 at 2:30 p.m. Please let me know if this appointment works for you, as this is Dr. Wilson's first available appointment.
>
> Thank you and have a nice day!

The ability to request an appointment via email is nice but hardly revolutionary. Although my need to see a doctor was not urgent, being scheduled for "the first available" appointment 7½ weeks from the day of the request was totally retrograde.

When he found out, Dr. Wilson was embarrassed about the long delay and sent a follow-up email saying he would double book and that I should call the office to schedule a time that was convenient for me. Eventually I saw my physician—after just 3½ weeks of waiting.

What is most troubling is that this is not an isolated event; indeed, a long delay is the usual experience for most Americans trying to schedule a doctor's appointment. Today the average time to get an appointment with a family physician is just under 20 days, the same amount of time it has been for the last 8 years.

Scheduling management is the first fundamental step in transforming a medical office or clinic. Each office's appointment book controls the most valuable asset of medicine: physicians' time. Time—and its allotment—is one of the most important, but often overlooked, aspects of transformation. In part it enhances office efficiency, and in part it communicates the transition to patient-centric care more strongly than any other transformative practice. Medical organizations that have successfully transformed their care have wrestled the office or clinic schedule away from physicians and front office staff. But although this is successful, wrestling that scheduling book away is not for the faint of heart. At Dean Clinic in Wisconsin, the management acknowledges that gaining control of scheduling "took a year and a half, and it burned out 2 of our medical directors."

Why is taking away the schedule so difficult? In part it embodies the seismic shift from a physician-centric to a patient-centric orientation of care. According to WESTMED CEO Simeon Schwartz, "the appointment book is the holy grail of transformation. . . . [For physicians] autonomy is synonymous with the scheduling book." It allows them to control when they work, how hard they work, and how often they work. When they control the scheduling book, physicians have various ways of manipulating their schedules to their liking. They block out times during the day when they do not want to see patients. They pad their schedules with visits from low-risk patients who have stable hypertension or angina, or with patients they like to talk to. They ensure that they always leave at 4:30 p.m. When physicians control the schedule, they ensure that they are busy—just not too busy.

Not only does physician-controlled scheduling allow physicians to be overly lenient with how they use their time, it is also totally inefficient. Each physician has different rules and preferences. Satisfying them consumes an enormous amount of the front-desk administrators' time. And if a patient needs to be seen urgently, perhaps that same day because of an accident, side effect of treatment, or some other event, it creates endless negotiations that waste the time of both the front office staff and the physician. Because so many individual scheduling rules change every week, it is almost impossible to make scheduling electronic, as no one can write such adaptable code. This makes it hard to implement electronic booking or create a smartphone app to allow patients to book appointments themselves. A senior physician at Dean Clinic describes the problem and inefficiencies:

> We had 400 different schedules in primary care with holds, blocks, rules for this and that—lunches and parties. Some doctors had rules that said they would not see anybody who was Spanish speaking or did not want two Spanish speaking patients in a row. An OB doctor said, unless it's a woman of child-bearing years who is in the situation where she could become pregnant, I don't want to see her. The rules for some doctors were thicker than the scheduling book for the year. We moved schedulers to a central location. We got them away from the physicians. We reduced the different types of appointments from 400 to 7.

Centralized appointments ensure that physicians are busy and that they are seeing both enough and the right types of patients. This is particularly important if physicians are paid a salary rather than fee-for-service, which might otherwise disincentive working hard and being productive.

A second advantage of centralized scheduling is the ability to adapt to the unexpected by allowing patients to see different providers as needed. It is important that physicians be able to see patients with urgent issues the same day in order to avoid unnecessary emergency room visits and the cascade of events and costs that follow. In multi-specialty group practices centralized scheduling also ensures that when a physician uncovers a serious problem, specialists can see that patient that same or the very next day.

A third advantage of centralized scheduling is that it actually frees up physicians' time. There has been increasing worry about a shortage of physicians in the United States, especially primary care physicians. Many have argued that introducing millions of patients into the health-care system through the universal coverage of the Affordable Care Act would lead to a physician shortage and longer waits. (Although there exists a widespread misconception that the ACA has lengthened time to see a physician, data indicate this has not happened.) In addition, physicians are constantly complaining about being overworked and not having enough time to devote to each patient. However, both of these complaints can be addressed, at least partially, through central-ized scheduling. Centralized scheduling has the tendency to reduce the number of office visits, primarily for patients who probably do not need to be seen as frequently as they are, such as patients whose blood pressure is stable and under control and those with well-controlled di-abetes or asthma. And when practices build in additional changes, such as having care managers call these patients or use telemonitoring to check on them remotely, care is actually streamlined. As one senior physician at Dean noted,

> If you started over and said, forget about the dollars, if the game was "What's the most efficient way to provide care, how would you do it?" We would not bring people into the office as often as we do. We just wouldn't.

> We would look at the data, we would look at the pieces of information we need, gathered by whomever or whatever technology—maybe it is their little blood pressure monitor that transmits over the phone into our system. And we could provide care less expensively ...

> Central scheduling allows us to get rid of some of these unnecessary ap-pointments and free up time for physicians and the team to see the sick and unstable patients who need to be seen.

Fourth, changing scheduling practices can be efficient in several ad-ditional ways. Rather than compartmentalizing offices, each separated by their own schedule, a clinic will have one overarching scheduling process. If one physician or practice is fully booked, the scheduling system will ensure that patients can set up appointments with another physician or nurse practitioner in the same practice or in an affiliated one.

Finally, centralized scheduling allows patients more options and control over how they receive care.

> Patient perception of access really improved. If you want to see Dr. Kaufmann, his next appointment is in 6 weeks, or you can see his partner in 2 days, or you can see his physician's assistant today. They [patients] may still take the option of seeing Dr. Kaufmann in 6 weeks, but we gave the decision to the patients. So the perception of access really just went up.

How is this first transformational practice operationalized? At WESTMED, centralization of scheduling was achieved by directing patient calls to a call center in North Carolina rather than to the doctor's office. When WESTMED initially centralized their scheduling, there were 25 scheduling "pods" specialized to different offices within the WESTMED system—the cardiologists assigned to 1 pod, the GI doctors to another, and the primary care physicians to a third. This "improvement" turned out to be inefficient. Each pod had specialized knowledge of the schedules of its own individual physician groups. Call center staff were not able to cross over to different pods. To fix this problem, WESTMED gave physician groups the chance to create their own scheduling rules and then converted those rules into an algorithm with branching logic that could be put on a computer for anyone in the North Carolina call center to use. The algorithm had a few thousand rules, of which 80% were general and only 20% were customized to specific specialist groups. Now any employee at the call center in North Carolina can follow the algorithm and schedule any type of appointment for any physician or office. Since automating its scheduling into an algorithm, WESTMED has begun the process of creating an online scheduling app that will allow patients to follow the same logic themselves, without having the North Carolina call center involved.

Beyond centralizing scheduling, many clinics and offices have transformed their care by switching to "open-access" scheduling. In essence, this means they leave a certain percentage of the physician and nurse practitioner appointments unscheduled at the start of every day. This practice was developed by the consultants Mark Murray and Catherine Tantau and promoted by the Institute for Healthcare Improvement (IHI). It has several steps. First, a clinic eliminates double booking, a technique used by doctors, like my own personal physician, Dr. Wilson, to squeeze patients in. As one health system manager explains, with open-access "we no longer double book, assuming that so many people aren't going to show that day." Essentially double booking ensures that patients wait a long time to see a physician or nurse and that even when they are seen, the visits are rushed. The physicians themselves also feel rushed and overwhelmed, running from patient to patient.

Second, to prevent chaos, clinics purposely and deliberately create open time on physicians' schedules: 20% to 50% of the appointment slots have no patients assigned to them at the start of the day. There is no consensus about the "right" amount of open appointment time. At one end of the spectrum, WESTMED keeps only 20% of physician appointments for open access. WESTMED management has found that having more than 20% open slots makes it hard to schedule future appointments for patients. Another expert advises having 30% of all appointments open, with even more open "on Mondays and after holidays when urgent-access visits are in high demand." At the other end of the spectrum, Murray and Tantau recommend filling only 30% of appointment time slots with patients, thereby keeping 70% of slots free at the start of the day.

Third, when patients call they are then given the opportunity to come in and see their personal physician at any of the available slots that very same day. If their personal physician has no time, then the patient should first be offered the next available appointment with their personal physician. If this is too far off or is at an inconvenient time for the patient, then an appointment with a colleague should be offered, and then finally a same-day appointment with the next available provider, whomever that may be.

These scheduling changes have many advantages. Patients are successfully seen the same day—or the day after—they call. Additionally, it actually reduces patient waiting times. Without double booking and with free appointment slots, patients can be brought quickly into exam rooms.

Although many physicians would perhaps fear an increase in patient no-show rates, the opposite actually occurs. Kaiser Permanente Mid-Atlantic, for example, saw a roughly 20% drop in no-show rates when it transitioned to open access, and IHI has reported practices with even greater declines. Patients who make a same-day appointment—say, to be seen in 3 hours—are much more likely to show up at the appointment. In addition, shorter wait times also incentivize patients not to miss an appointment.

Another widely reported advantage is happier physicians and staff. It is easy—and satisfying—to tell a patient who urgently calls that, "The doctor can see you in 2 hours." Interestingly, open-access, centralized scheduling also reduces the time physicians spend trying to negotiate their schedules to accommodate patients. Furthermore, it reduces "leakage." Because they can be seen right away, patients do not try to go to other physicians—or if they do, they will first try their specialist instead.

Finally, open-access scheduling reduces the use of emergency rooms and urgent care facilities. When a physician or nurse practitioner can see a patient the same day, there is much less need to send a patient to the emergency room. Fewer emergency room visits almost invariably mean fewer hospitalizations. Main Line Oncology outside Philadelphia perfectly illustrates this point. To better address the side effects of chemotherapy, Main Line's CEO John Sprandio created algorithms for managing nausea, vomiting, diarrhea, insomnia, and other common complications based on guidelines created by the National Cancer Institute. These guidelines specify what questions to ask patients, what medications might be prescribed to ameliorate the symptoms, and when the symptoms are sufficiently severe that the patient needs to be seen by a physician. Nurses then use these algorithms when answering patient calls. If the algorithm indicates a patient needs to be seen urgently, there are appointment slots for both nurse practitioners and oncologists that are kept unscheduled. Sprandio keeps 30% of daily appointments open. Since adopting open access scheduling, Main Line has seen more than a 50% decline in emergency room visits in just over 6 years.

Regardless of its many benefits, there are some barriers to implementing centralized scheduling. For example, it is difficult to assuage physicians' fears that there will be too many unfilled appointments and a resulting drop in revenue. This fear is commonplace, despite the fact that most organizations report that it does not occur. Indeed, by having fewer no-shows and fewer front office staff, many practices end up being more efficient and seeing increased revenues and margins. As the experiences of many transformed practices show, shifting control of scheduling takes both time and a fair amount of good will, but it will ultimately add to the strength of a physician governance system.

Changing scheduling practices by moving from a physician-centric to a patient-centric model may be the most tangible way a physician group can communicate to patients that they really are committed to enhancing patient experience. Organizations and providers should also be on board, as this change can increase revenue and employee satisfaction.

PRACTICE 2: REGISTERING AND ROOMING PATIENTS

Is there anything more annoying than going to a physician, physical therapy, or CT scan appointment and having to fill out, by hand, all that paperwork? Over and over you find yourself writing down your address, your next of kin, your current insurance company, a review of potential problems with your heart, thyroid, lungs, and every other organ system; your medications, allergies, any changes in health status; and whatever else the physician's office or hospital thinks they need. Occasionally you forget your insurance card, which must be photocopied. This process seems repetitive, unproductive, and fraught with errors. Even after registering, you wait and wait. Finally, a nurse escorts you to the examination room, where you wait again until the harried physician comes in. Nothing seems so annoying and wasteful as the registration and rooming processes at physician offices and other medical facilities.

Improving registration will remove this patient frustration, save money relegated to office staff, and offer insight into patient flow. Changing the rooming process can also be a highly effective way to ensure that patients receive the basic, effective tests and treatments they need, such as colonoscopies and flu vaccines, also known as closing gaps in care.

ChenMed of Florida offers one solution for this frustrating patient registration problem. Based in Miami, Florida, ChenMed is a family-owned collection of primary care practices that mainly serve low- to moderate-income elderly patients largely under contracts with Medicare Advantage insurers. They have recently expanded, with new practices in Louisville, Virginia Beach, Richmond, and several other locations. Chris Chen, the son of the founder, is currently the CEO. At 6-foot-3, with slicked-back, jet-black hair and a penchant for dressing like a Wall Street executive—complete with expensive suits and cuff links—Chris Chen does not immediately seem to fit into his organization's more Spartan, clinical settings. Still, this Taiwanese American cardiologist proudly shows off his clinics, particularly the "ChenMed card" that each patient has. Each card encodes a variety of patient information, and on the back is printed each patient's EKG—a recording of the heart's electrical conductivity. Once a patient flashes his card near a radio frequency ID (RFID) reader, the receptionist's computer screen displays his picture and name, enabling the receptionist to address him personally. With the card there is no need for the receptionist to ask who he is or which physician he is coming to see. The ChenMed card also gives the receptionist instantaneous access to all the patient's old information—address, next of kin, insurance company, list of past medical problems, allergies, current medications, and so forth. The patient can quickly verify any information without the need to—yet again—complete any forms. Lastly, the flash of the card alerts a health aide, equipped with an iPad, that the patient has just checked in and is waiting. As Dr. Chen says,

> Patients come in here, scan their card, and are checked in. Done. Then two things occur. Number one, the person at the front desk sees the face pop up and can say, "Everything looks great, Mr. So-and-so. Great, have a seat." The receptionist greets the patient by name, [so] you immediately create that relationship.
>
> Then, in real time the systems check insurance eligibility. So it just makes it convenient. No more insurance cards. No more Medicare cards. Patients bring one card—our card—and scan it.

What Chen is probably most proud of is the way in which ChenMed ensures that patients actually keep their cards and reliably bring them to appointments:

> We tell people, "You need to carry this card. Don't lose it." How do we do that? We tell patients their life depends on it. . . . How do we ensure we are not lying to them? If the patient had syncope and fainted, they are rushed to the hospital emergency room, they have an old EKG on the back of the card to compare to the one taken at the hospital.

Understandably the thought that their lives depend on these cards has resonated with patients—and so most carry their ChenMed card with them at all times.

Certify, a privately held company, has gone further than ChenMed in transforming the registration process. Marc Potash, CEO and founder, began developing his technology far from healthcare, in the world of karate and parking garages. As a chiropractic student, Marc taught karate. But he had a problem: How to regularly bill 800 students without inputting the billing information manually every month? This was back in 1997, before PayPal, Venmo, and all the other Web-enabled applications. To solve his problem Potash developed the first Web-based billing application. His next challenge was applying his technology to parking garages, specifically linking the automatic billing and payment information with the gates at 280 different garages in different cities so that when someone paid their monthly bill, the gate would open. Then in 2010 Potash turned his attention to healthcare.

Certify uses 2-factor biometrics to register and authenticate a patient. With a fingerscan and a picture of the patient's face, the system can identify a specific patient. The first-time relevant information is either pulled from the patient's electronic health record (EHR) or the patient inputs her name, address, next of kin, insurance, allergies, and all the other information. Like many smartphone apps, Certify can take a picture of the patient's insurance card and input the info directly into the system—no photo-copying of the insurance card ever again. At subsequent visits, the information appears, and the patient simply confirms it or makes revisions. Any specific forms the practice or hospital needs completed come up electronically and are integrated into the patient's EHR. This registration can occur on a laptop, a specially programmed tablet, or at a specially designed kiosk in a physician's office or hospital—much like registering at an airline for a flight, except that there is no confirmation number or frequent-flyer number to be punched in; it is all done literally by touch.

The system then does several things that benefit physician practices and hospitals. First, it confirms the patient's identity through 2 biometrics, which significantly reduces patient-generated fraud. Anyone trying to pose as another person to scam insurers or obtain narcotics or other drugs from emergency room physicians are detected: no one can register with the same fingerprints and face as Sam Smith and then subsequently as Sam Jones.

Second, having a unique biometric identifier eliminates duplicate records—not a trivial problem at hospitals and other systems.

Third, Certify has created a way of integrating many legacy systems. Many facilities have different inpatient and outpatient EHRs that do not interact, but Certify has merged them so that the information from each system is available in one place. Physician practices that merge may be using different EHRs; Certify can grab the information from the disparate systems and make it available. In this sense, legacy systems are no longer a barrier to interoperability.

Fourth, the system is also HIPAA compliant and can pull up all relevant records in the office or hospital—or, indeed, at any of the physician offices or hospitals linked to Certify. This allows a physician to see the note from a patient's recent ER visit or the record from a hospitalization. Currently Certify has 22,000 physicians using its system through physician offices and hospitals, and is integrated with many of the leading EHRs and practice-management systems, including EPIC, Cerner, McKesson, Athena, Allscripts, eClinical Works, GE Centricity, and others. As the Certify network grows, the electronic information from institutions that can populate a patient's record also grows.

Fifth, by linking to a tag issued to the patient or patient's cell phone through ultra-high-frequency radio frequency ID (UHF RFID), patients and visitors can be tracked as they move about. This allows a hospital to measure wait times and inform patients and visitors how long they have waited. It also enhances security by ensuring they are not going to floors or other places they should not.

Finally, because it relies on biometrics, a patient who arrives in the emergency room unconscious can still be identified and their relevant past medical information called up in Certify.

The Certify system is multilingual, providing screens in Spanish, Mandarin, and other languages. Because the system is linked to insurers as well, it eliminates sticker shock months after a visit. Certify can provide a patient, at registration, with an estimated financial impact of the visit, the amount applied to deductible, the co-pay, and any other charges. And Certify can process a payment seamlessly at the end of the visit to a credit card that has been swiped at registration or stored on the system.

This is just the beginning of the advantages of Certify. By having a fraud-proof patient identification, authentication, and registration system and by linking to many EHRs, practice-management systems, and other health vendors, Certify can seamlessly connect a patient to pharmacies so that medications can be ordered from the physician office and delivered when the patient arrives at home. It can automatically print or electronically deliver a schedule to a patient who has multiple visits at a facility.

Certify can produce savings by reducing fraud, registration and other personnel costs, and by ensuring more complete EHRs. For instance, Certify is currently being installed at all of University of Pittsburgh Medical Center's (UPMC) 22 hospitals, which employ a total of 3,500 physicians. According to Ed McCallister, UPMC's chief information officer,

> Certify gives us the ability for interoperability, enabling us to integrate all of our legacy systems so we can have all of our patient data available in one place.
>
> By implementing Certify, we are eliminating duplicate records, reducing patient and physician identity fraud, reallocating front desk registration staff as well as the many other types of savings we are witnessing. Certify results in greater efficiencies, extremely high patient satisfaction and potential for millions of dollars in savings.

The University of Pennsylvania Health System is also trying Certify as a pilot.

Another benefit of Certify is that it enhances the patient experience. Not only is the annoyance of repeatedly writing basic information on paper forms eliminated, but the instantaneous presentation of patient information—name and picture, insurance status, and who they have an appointment with—also allows for personalized interactions between the receptionist and patient. Both are a move toward making a visit to the physician more attentive to the patient's needs, with fewer errors and less staff time.

Such registration methods also help physicians and offices improve patient flow. When a patient registers via a card or biometric, as at ChenMed, a time stamp is created, allowing the office to measure wait times. How long did the patient have to sit in the waiting room before being escorted to a room? How long was the patient in the room before a physician or other clinician entered for the exam? How long was the clinician-patient interaction? At Chen Med, such questions are easily answered through the use of card-triggered time stamps:

> The card provides a time stamp, so we know exactly what time the patient left. So we can definitively say our average wait time was 16 minutes from the time they scanned the card to getting into the exam room and the doctor walking in.

It is certainly possible to track registration manually, but automating this process with an RFID-enabled card makes it immediate, seamless, less error prone, and more difficult for offices to cover up undesirable delays and long waits. Ultimately, this data helps providers determine where there are consistent bottlenecks in their delivery of care. Providers can then develop effective solutions to facilitate patient flow.

EVEN MORE IMPORTANT than registration for bringing about transformation is rooming. Rooming is when patients are taken from the waiting room to the exam room—a seemingly simple and not very important step. But many practices have begun transforming what used to be a largely social encounter, with the recording of height, weight, and blood pressure, into a valuable medical intervention.

Practices are increasingly being held accountable for meeting specific quality measures, such as ensuring patients have received the age-appropriate cancer screenings, ensuring blood pressure is controlled, making sure diabetic patients have their hemoglobin A1c in the right range, and seeing that patients with high cholesterol are on the right medications. Care gaps occur when patients do not have these recommended services. In order to ensure such gaps are closed, electronic registration systems such as those used by ChenMed or Certify are linked to a patient's EHR and automatically bring up a list of the deficiencies in recommended care. The person rooming the patient is empowered to ensure all recommended care is ordered—all before the physician or another clinician even enters the room.

Transformed physician offices such as VillageMD, WESTMED, Dean Clinic, and ChenMed have adopted very similar rooming systems. VillageMD has 9 locations, with 50 primary care physicians. They have licensed practical nurses and medical assistants (LPNs and MAs) do the rooming. When the patient is registered, a nurse or medical assistant is notified of their arrival, and a list of recommended care items that have not occurred is presented electronically. The LPN or MA greets the registered patient and escorts them from the waiting room to the exam room. The LPNs and MAs are empowered to close as many care gaps as possible, off-loading from the physician as much of the nonmedical work as possible. They order all the mammograms, DXA scans for assessing bone density, and other required screening tests; they administer required immunizations, such as flu and pneumonia vaccines; and they conduct depression and fall screening tests. At VillageMD, the LPNs and MAs will even complete a brief history to focus the patient's time with the physician.

ChenMed employs a similar system but uses medical assistants instead of nurses. As Chris Chen explains:

> When you scan the card, the electronic medical system says, "Oh there's a patient in the waiting room," alerting the team. The health aide then goes out and picks up the patient and then immediately opens up what tests they have due. With the card the health aide can see if the patient is due for a hemoglobin A1c test, a mammogram, or a DXA scan—all of these things.

Thus, everything a normal doctor would do in terms of health maintenance and care gaps is done before the doctor walks in the room. We turn medical assistants into physician extenders because they have a tablet that creates customized screens for them to follow as the patient checks in.

VillageMD has created a 15-page "Rooming Guidelines" booklet with a 32-page addendum to both train LPNs and MAs and to use as a resource for consultation. The guidelines identify specific activities that need to be performed for patients based on age, sex, and presenting symptoms. This prephysician preparation covers not just vital signs but also medication reconciliation, age, and sex-specific exams such as fall assessments and cervical cancer screening. The guidelines even have disease-specific assessments for patients with asthma and other chronic conditions as well as disease-specific education for patients. They allow physicians to spend as much time as possible providing those cognitive and diagnostic services that only doctors can do. The guidelines also ensure that rooming is done the same way by every LPN and MA at all 9 VillageMD locations. This standardization in turn ensures that any assistant can help any physician, and that when a medical assistant is sick or on vacation, the flow of the office is not disrupted.

In these transformed offices the LPN or MA is also expected to alert physicians of any abnormal physical, laboratory, or other findings so the physician can address them. For instance, many practices have their MAs list all abnormal results, such as blood pressure and weight, at the top of each patient's chart, thereby alerting physicians of any issues that can then be efficiently addressed during the office visit without the physician needing to compare today's blood pressure or weight to the reading from the previous office visit.

Linking rooming with ensuring recommended care is ordered, medications are reconciled, and some disease education has occurred leads to increased efficiencies and cost reductions. However, the innovation in rooming affects employees in different ways. Typically, it takes rooming away from registered nurses, giving this task instead to LPNs and medical assistants. Nurses may resist this change. They often enjoy and receive positive feedback from patient interaction during rooming. However, having registered nurses room patients is inefficient. There are other, more valuable ways for nurses to interact with patients, such as managing the ones with serious illnesses. As one Dean administrator explained,

> It's not appropriate for a [registered nurse, RN] to be rooming patients. [But] it's their favorite part of the job, so we really were disrupting things. Now the [medical assistants] do the rooming. The LPNs and the unit clerks have their role, and the RNs, based on their licensing, have their own role: based on their licensing work, it's teaching, it's triaging.

Conversely, comprehensive and consistent rooming practices move the responsibility for closing gaps from physicians alone to a team. At VillageMD this change has improved the job satisfaction of LPNs, MAs, and physicians. Taking away the responsibility to close care gaps from physicians and also having the rooming LPNs and MAs alert physicians to any abnormal results frees up time during the actual office visit. The physicians find that they are spending almost no time fumbling through records, looking for the last hemoglobin A1c or spirometry result; instead, they can spend more time literally looking at patients and discussing meaningful health issues. This effectively lengthens and enhances the physician-patient interaction.

Such value is placed on closing care gaps that medical organizations often use the performance of rooming practices in formal job evaluations. At WESTMED, the medical assistants' job evaluations are primarily based on how well they close care gaps. Similar to how physician performance is evaluated based on the fulfillment of standard quality metrics, rooming staff are measured by using graphs of the number and percent of care gaps they have closed, information they receive via report cards. As part of its rooming guidelines, VillageMD also has a "competency assessment" form that covers everything from professionalism, communication, and patient care to hand-washing skills, vital signs, medications, computer skills, and critical thinking.

Thus, changing the registration and rooming processes of care can lead to more efficient and improved care in 3 main ways. First, it allows

LPNs and MAs, rather than highly trained registered nurses, to room patients. Second, it empowers LPNs and MAs to participate in meaningful medical management; in particular, by standardizing the rooming process, LPNs and MAs ensure all recommended care is systematically addressed. Finally, it frees up physicians' time, allowing them to focus on more meaningful health issues with patients during the office visit.

Registration and rooming seem like such an unimportant part of the office visit that many providers often do not realize that they could be part of transforming the delivery of care. Yet many of the leading practices have focused on improving these steps to add value. Electronic registration enhances patient satisfaction both by eliminating paperwork and by improving the efficiency of front office staff; it also reduces costly duplicate records and fraud. Similarly, entrusting rooming to LPNs or MAs who are empowered and expected to close care gaps and alert physicians of abnormalities ensures that recommended care is performed consistently, systematically, and efficiently.

PRACTICE 3: MEASURING PHYSICIAN PERFORMANCE

Almost every week I get a call from a personal or family friend that goes something like this:

> A few days ago I called my dad in Miami. He sounded confused, and his speech was slurred. I panicked and called his primary care physician. When I called my dad back about 30 minutes later, he was fine; he was alert, and his speech was almost back to normal.
>
> What should I do? Is this his brain? Who should I call? Do I stick with his primary care doctor, or do I need a neurologist? Who is the best neurologist in Miami that I can get him to see? Where is the best place for him to be treated?

The implied request is that I will identify one of the top neurologists and one of the best hospitals in Miami to treat or prevent transitory ischemic attacks and strokes and ensure that my friend's father gets an appointment.

Truth be told, finding the best doctor or hospital in a city—that is, being able to objectively evaluate physician and hospital performance—is a problem everyone faces, laymen and physicians alike. Indeed, most physicians know very little about their own performance. They think they are practicing superb medicine—how else could they get up every morning and treat patients? But are they really? Most physicians do not have the comparative data to really know how well they are practicing. Objective data for comparing physician quality is exceedingly limited; instead, everyone in the healthcare system—physicians included—tends to rely on word of mouth, *US News & World Report*, or local organizations' doctor lists. These rankings are more rumor and gossip than data-driven, objective measures.

One of the oft-repeated catchphrases of healthcare performance improvement is that "if you can't measure it, you can't manage it."* In medicine today it is not that we *can't* measure performance but rather that we *don't* systematically measure and compare it. And because we do not measure it, we do not report it, and as a consequence, people cannot learn from the data or use them to improve.

---

*Interestingly, this quote is frequently—and, it turns out, mistakenly—attributed to either the famed business consultant Peter Drucker or quality expert W. Edwards Deming. As Robert Berenson and a few others have pointed out, neither Drucker nor Deming actually believed that "if you can't measure it, you can't manage it." Indeed, both knew that there were important aspects of organizations that could not be measured but had to be managed. Both emphasized that it was not possible to measure personal interactions and culture, yet both are critical to an organization's success and had to be managed.

In a 1990 interview, Drucker even went so far as to disavow the absolute power of measurement when discussing corporate leadership, saying,

Your first role ... is the personal one, it is the relationship with people, the development of mutual confidence, the identification of people, the creation of community. This is something only you can do. ... It cannot be measured or easily defined. But it is not only a key function. It is the one only you can perform.

Similarly, according to the W. Edwards Deming Institute the full quote is: "*It is wrong to suppose* that if you can't measure it, you can't manage it—a costly myth" (emphasis added).

For whatever reason, over the years that quote has been shortened and remolded to fit the argument for the necessity of measurement in management.

Thus, a third transformational practice is measuring and reporting performance data and using it to improve the quality of care. Every office, hospital, or healthcare system that has truly transformed care has devoted significant resources to measuring physician and health system performance and to reporting the results of those measurements to physicians and other stakeholders. Furthermore, the provider organizations that have had the most success do not just measure the performance of their physicians; they extend their rigorous performance analyses to every worker in their system in order to get a clear assessment of collective performance.

Truthfully, many physicians are—or, at least until recently, have been—reluctant to engage in this performance measurement, especially if the results are made public. Physicians raise a myriad of by now well-rehearsed objections: "There are no data"; "The data are flawed"; "My patients are [pick your descriptor: sicker, poorer, less educated, less compliant], so bad performance is not my fault." And on and on. But office practices, hospitals, and health systems that are truly committed to transformation ignore these views—or, more accurately, spend the time to rebut them (see pages 49–50)—and institutionalize systematic performance measurement and reporting back to clinicians.

The first challenge to actually measure performance is determining the metrics on which physicians should be assessed. Even at this stage there are 5 additional subchallenges obtaining: (1) well-validated metrics; (2) metrics with sufficient numbers of patients that the results are meaningful; (3) metrics that can be risk-adjusted to reflect true differences in patients' condition; (4) metrics for which the office, hospital, health system, or payer can provide timely data; and (5) physician buy-in and active participation in the performance-assessment program. These 5 challenges are not insurmountable, but overcoming them does require an active, deliberate, and sustained effort.

In selecting the metrics, organizations should begin with uncontroversial metrics that physicians already accept—or at least cannot ignore. One such set of metrics is the traditional HEDIS—Healthcare Effectiveness Data and Information Set—measures. HEDIS now has 81 rigorously vetted measures that are used by the government, insurers, and payers to assess performance on quality. Nevertheless, most are process measures that physicians often balk at or dismiss as irrelevant.

In addition, there are several other performance measures that can be used. CMS and private payers often use other metrics to rate hospitals and health systems, such as emergency room utilization, readmission rates, and, for some patients, mortality. Payers are increasingly using HEDIS and their own metrics to award bonuses or to adjust reimbursement levels. Because money is already linked to these measures, physicians acknowledge them as important, even if they are also view them as unpleasant.

Perhaps the best way for medical organizations to select metrics is to not select them at all. Many practices, hospitals, and health systems have put metric selection back into the hands of physicians and used this as an effective way to create physician buy-in. If physicians themselves select the metrics on which they will be evaluated, they can hardly object to being evaluated on them; indeed, including physicians in this process affords them the level of agency and control they deserve, while transforming their position relative to the program. Instead of complaining about something that is imposed upon them from on high, physicians can take ownership of the process and hold themselves and their system accountable for results they have affirmatively deemed important and meaningful. Including physicians may take more time and effort, but it will frequently avert management headaches born of physician intransigence, while also improving the overall efficacy of performance measurement.

Physician participation in measurement selection can be combined with other mechanisms to facilitate physician buy-in to the performance-measurement process. One approach is to link physician pay or bonuses to their actual performance. This tends to better engage physicians in metric selection. Yet another approach is to require physicians to participate in performance-improvement activities. For instance, WESTMED requires their clinical departments to create at least one department-wide quality improvement or cost-reduction project of their own choosing each year. Although physicians might be reluctant at first, their participation can lead them to accept and affirm their measure of quality as well as related activities, such as the standardization of care processes. As one WESTMED cardiologist explained:

> So we come up with things that we think need to be improved. . . . This
> year's project is making sure patients who have valves have antibiotics
> discussed with them. . . . Everybody's really trying to follow the guide-
> lines and doing evidence-based medicine. So I think we're all on the
> same page.

Despite being exasperated with the process, this cardiologist was very
happy with WESTMED and acknowledged that the previous year's
care-improvement activity that focused on making management of
atrial fibrillation more standardized did seem to work and enhance
consistency and quality.

At Hoag Orthopedic Institute, a joint venture between a nonprofit
hospital and a group of orthopedic surgeons in Orange County, California, the physicians developed the metrics used to assess all hip and
knee replacements. They included several hard data points, such as the
rates of surgical site infections, blood clots, and 30-day readmission as
well as patient-reported outcomes, including the degree to which patients were pain-free, whether they could resume playing sports, and
their overall quality of life, each of which was measured several times
over the 9 months after the operation. These metrics, as it turned out,
were also meaningful for patients.

Similarly, there are important objective measures in oncology that
should be used for evaluating performance. These include providing
a designated "preferred" chemotherapy—one proven in clinical trials
and certified by professional organizations—for a cancer, providing
the right dose intensity without inappropriate dose reductions of the
chemotherapy, and providing the number of emergency room visits
and hospitalizations for side effects after chemotherapy administration. Other measures that are also relevant include patient-reported
outcomes, such as frequency of nausea and vomiting as well as pain
levels. One of the physicians at Dean describes his experience with performance measurement this way:

> To be honest with you, there are a lot of departments where we don't
> have great data. But primary care, cardiology, cardiovascular surgery,
> and orthopedics are probably the big ones where we have a lot of data.
> For instance, the percent of your diabetic patients whose hemoglobin

A1c is controlled to goal, is under 7%. The percent of your ischemic vascular disease patients who have had their LDL measured in their last interval of time. We use data sets from HEDIS and the Wisconsin Collaborative on Healthcare Quality.

How should the data be risk adjusted? There are several risk-adjustment methodologies that could be used on the data, though none can perfectly account for all the variability between patients. One option is to adopt the risk-adjustment methods used by Medicare and other payers. Because these methodologies are actually used to influence reimbursement and bonus payments to physicians and health systems, it is hard for physicians to object to them. Including the physicians who are to be evaluated in this process has another advantage: although physicians might complain to administrators that their patients are sicker and that is why their performance is not as good as others, it is much harder to make this "reverse Lake Wobegon" claim to physician colleagues. Your colleagues know your patients cannot be sicker than their patients. This often means that risk adjustment itself can be dispensed with—or if done, the endless discussion of how much variability it accounts for can be short circuited. As one physician explains,

> My colleagues in my department don't buy the fact that my patients are a little bit older than their patients and that my patients are a little bit sicker. They are kind of like, "I'm taking care of the same stuff, the same kinds of patients, that you are. Give me a break claiming your performance isn't as good because of your patients."

Annual performance is well-nigh worthless. After a year it is impossible for physicians to relate their performance to particular patients. The best offices, hospitals, and health systems use real-time performance data; physicians can see their performance up through the previous day. If real-time reporting is too complex an endeavor for a practice, even monthly reporting is useful.

After the metrics are defined, risk adjusted, collected, and put into a presentable format, the big question is what to do with them. There are numerous approaches regarding how and how often to report back the data to physicians and other staff. There is insufficient research to confidently say what constitutes the optimal approach. Nevertheless, physician groups and health systems have successfully tried different approaches, and there are important lessons.

Initially many health systems and physician offices provided the data to physicians in a blinded manner. For example, a physician would be shown a bar graph of his or her performance relative to others in the group but with the other names blanked out or converted into a number (see Figure 4.1, page 227). Many offices, hospitals, or health systems that used anonymous reporting of performance found that it did not improve performance, so they adopted unblinded performance feedback instead. They listed by name all the physicians in a group, typically a department like cardiology or a specific clinical site, who were being evaluated. The physicians could then see their own performance relative to their known colleagues. Systems made this change with trepidation. As one health system administrator put it, "We had heartburn about listing physicians' names on the internal practice performance evaluation." But the unblinded reporting of performance typically does produce positive performance change.

Hummy Song, one of my colleagues at the Wharton School, and her research team quantitatively studied the impact of sharing personally identifiable performance data on the comparative performance of emergency room physicians at Kaiser facilities. They showed that the lower-ranking physicians' performance improved and did so within a few quarters. Indeed, according to Professor Song, sharing identifiable performance data among the emergency room physicians was "associated with a 10.7% improvement in physician productivity and no significant reduction in service quality."

Identifiable release of performance data relies on the behavioral economics principle of peer comparisons and the basic human drive not to be embarrassed in front of people you know and interact with regularly. More importantly, there are 3 specific ways that the release of unblinded performance data can generate changes in physician behavior. At its simplest, unblinded data changes performance because physicians are super-competitive. Since their adolescence physicians have been subjected to an intense Darwinian selection process in which they have had to perform at the top of their college classes to get into medical school, at the top of their medical school to get into a highly reputable internship and residency programs, and at the top of their residency class to get the best specialty fellowships and jobs. Releasing identifiable performance data harnesses this competitive tendency in order to improve the actual practice of medicine. As one physician said,

> Most of the physicians are Type A personalities . . . where it is embarrassing if you are not at the top level of performance compared to your colleagues. There are not a whole lot of excuses. So there is nowhere to hide. And most of the physicians strive to improve.

A second mechanism by which identifiable data improves performance is through the sharing of knowledge. Physicians can see which of their colleagues are excelling and find out what these positive outliers do differently that might improve their own performance. One physician remembers the experience of first receiving his performance data:

> As soon as the system started generating data, I remember my own thought was, "This is silly. I know I am going to do great on this performance review." And then I saw my data. Holy cow, not nearly as good as I thought. Knowing that made me realize, "Hey we've got to be sharing this data." But more importantly it made me ask, "Who is doing the best?" I needed to look at that person and say, "What are you doing? How do you do it so well?"

Dr. Loftus reports the same phenomenon at Kaiser Permanente Mid-Atlantic:

> We use the physicians' names, and we talk about the fact that the opportunity here is for physicians to go down the hallway to their colleague, who is showing up better than they are, and have that conversation. . . . You also start to see changes in performance because the doctors are having those hallway conversations or behind-the-office-door conversations with their colleagues that do better.

Some physician practices and health systems systematize this data-sharing process. They hold sessions where different physicians share what they do that improves their performance. For instance, when Blue Cross Blue Shield of Massachusetts introduced the Alternative Quality

Contracts (AQC) that incentivized physicians to improve quality and make them accountable for total cost of care, they provided the physician groups with reports, established formal mechanisms for the groups to see each other's performance, and, more importantly, share best practices. The clinical leaders from the various groups discussed innovations in care delivery and what they deemed to be their best interventions. In addition, care managers, pharmacy user groups, and others came together for the sharing of more technical aspects of care. Dana Gelb Safran, chief performance measurement and improvement officer at Blue Cross Blue Shield of Massachusetts (BCBSMA), believes that a multifaceted program for sharing data and best practices has been a key to both the success of physician groups in the AQC program and to transforming the payer-provider relationship toward increased collaboration:

> A few times a year we bring the clinical leadership of the physician groups together at what we call our HEC forum. The first pillar of these forums involves a significant amount of data and information sharing from Mass Blue Cross and Blue Shield to the providers. We share data and performance reports such as the monthly claims data and about 60 different kinds of analytic reports that are given to groups on a regular basis—sometimes daily, monthly, or quarterly. Second, we pull in our expertise as a payer—including a multidisciplinary AQC support team with clinicians, performance improvement experts, and managers—to meet the clinical leadership of each organization and discuss their performance data and what they have tried so far, what's working and what's not, and to consult on new approaches to make further improvements.
>
> The third pillar is the best-practice sharing. Several times a year, we bring together the clinic leadership to discuss interesting innovations in care delivery and design. We have outside speakers, but one of these forums is always dedicated to groups sharing with each other their best innovations and learning from each other.

Hummy Song found that the Kaiser emergency room physicians who were performing less well asked those who were performing better what changes they could make to improve. As she put it, the "change [in performance] is accompanied by top-ranked physicians—whose identities are no longer anonymous—being asked by their colleagues to share their best practices." This study confirms reports from various physician organizations of the importance of releasing identifiable data to facilitate the sharing of best practices, thereby improving overall performance.

Some health systems have adopted yet a third mechanism for using the unblinded performance data to improve care: physician coaching. As a Dean management professional explains,

> We unblinded patient satisfaction data. And not just for the doctors, but for the entire organization. So anybody who works at Dean—anybody—can see Dr. X's patient satisfaction scores. That was a huge battle among the physician community. But we added a physician shadow coaching program. Now we have had consecutive quarters of improvement.

Other physician groups choose not to share the identifiable data internally among physicians; instead, they have one of their physician leaders personally meet with each physician to review their performance data. During this meeting they also compare the individual physician's data to aggregate data. The underlying philosophy at these sites is that using identifiable data raises physicians' hackles, generating negative push-back. At Hoag Orthopedic Institute, Dr. Robert Gorab, Hoag's chief medical officer, meets annually with each physician to personally review all their data. Dr. James Caillouette, Hoag's chief strategy officer, explains the group's philosophy:

> We do not use data as a weapon, because when you come at a surgeon using data as a weapon, you get push-back. Surgeons are notoriously difficult. And if you identify the surgeon's performance publicly, it turns ugly. You don't need to go unblinded. Instead, leadership personally reviews performance with each individual surgeon on the yearly review of report cards.

Hoag does publicly identify physicians who are performing well so others can learn from them. But, as they say,

We are not shaming low performers. If we see somebody who is better, we will say in an open session of our meeting with joint surgeons or whomever: "Hey, so-and-so is doing this, none of the rest of us can do this, we should look at doing this."

At Hoag, each physician is compared to the aggregate of all the MDs. Additionally, surgeons' case costs are compared to the Medicare DRG, its fixed payment amount for specific services. This encourages physicians to think about whether they are breaking even with Medicare, "a metric that is necessary to the long-term sustainability of the enterprise."

Advocate Health Care, the largest integrated delivery system in Illinois, with 12 hospitals and over 6,300 affiliated physicians, uses both identifiable performance reports and personal meetings with physicians to circulate their performance measurement data. Each physician can look up on the computer in real time how they compare to colleagues in both their department and geographic area on various measures, such as hemoglobin A1c control or 30-day hospital readmission rates. Additionally, every month Advocate sends out a report that includes each physician's performance data. To ensure they look at and understand the reports, each physician also meets with an Advocate representative to review the data. Meetings with primary care physicians take place on a monthly basis, while meetings with specialty physicians take place on a quarterly basis. These meetings are required for ongoing participation in the clinically integrated network. They are used to identify barriers and solve problems that will facilitate performance improvement. Performance on these metrics are linked to annual physician incentive compensation. To ensure that physicians do not resent the time commitment, Advocate actually compensates the physicians for each meeting as if they were seeing a patient. This ensures that physicians do not lose income by spending time on data review.

Performance measurement and feedback to physicians is critical to transformation. By now there are many well-accepted performance metrics and risk-adjustment methodologies available. Physicians can help affirm those that are available and can also develop their own. Transformed practices and groups have found that releasing the performance data in an unblinded manner to fellow physicians enhances performance. It allows physicians to know how well they are performing against both national benchmarks and their own colleagues. Disseminating unblinded data also allows physicians to identify outstanding performers and learn what they are doing that may improve their own performance.

PRACTICE 4: STANDARDIZING PATIENT CARE

On a recent Monday afternoon, Jocelyn Wolf took her 2 children, ages 8 and 5, to their pediatrician's office for their annual preschool physical examinations. Her pediatrician's office is the best.The pediatricians routinely make the coveted list of DC's top doctors in the glossy *Washingtonian* magazine. On this occasion, the children happened to be seen by 2 different pediatricians. Personalities aside, the children ended up having 2 very different exams in the same practice. Although both had the usual height, weight, BMI, blood pressure, and heart rate checks, the rest of the history and advice diverged—and not because the children had different health states. One pediatrician asked the 5-year-old boy about "organized activities," which seemed to be an inquiry into how much physical activity he engaged in; nothing about "organized activity" or the extent of physical activity was asked of the 8-year-old girl. Additionally, the 5-year-old boy was scheduled for a nurse-administered eye examination, while the 8-year-old girl was not, even though the American Association of Pediatrics recommends vision and hearing screening for both 5- and 8-year-olds. Conversely, the girl received advice to drink three 8-ounce glasses of milk each day, advice that was not offered to the 5-year-old boy. And both children received advice about seasonal allergies—but different advice. Both pediatricians advised taking an over-the-counter drug, but one merely suggested it while the other was insistent and strongly recommended pairing it with a steroid spray. Ironically, the nurse assigned to perform the 5-year-old's eye exam never performed one, as it was not part of her routine tasks.

Unjustified variation in care practices has been a major issue in American healthcare since at least the early 1970s, when several scientific articles documented variations in practices between adjacent New England towns. Since then the *Dartmouth Atlas* has become a treasure trove of examples of how medical practices, procedures like prostate surgery and mastectomy, hospitalization rates, and a myriad of other services vary between neighboring hospitals, cities, counties, and states.

Eliminating unjustified variation in care through standardization, with the ability to customize to particular patients, is an important component of transforming care. This step brings up the bottom by improving quality, reducing errors, and saving time and money because physicians and nurses do not have to work out all the details of care each time they see a patient. Instead, care of common problems, which usually consume a huge proportion of health providers' time, becomes a kind of muscle memory.

John Sprandio oversees a group of 9 oncologists in suburban Philadelphia. Within the group, they initially

> had 4 different ways to treating stomatitis—the mouth sores that come from certain types of chemotherapy. It required the nurses to remember which doctor preferred which oral care regimen and specific mouth wash treatment. And if a physician's patient got the wrong treatment, there was always someone who was upset.

Sprandio sat everyone down, and they worked out one way they would all use to treat stomatitis. It took a few meetings, but they eventually agreed, and created a standardized order set. Since then, all the oncologists have followed the same protocol, and the nurses no longer have to remember 4 different regimens; they just follow one. The group did the same with prophylactic medications for nausea and vomiting. Given the cost difference between drugs, they aimed for the most effective generic drugs available. This allowed them to have a single protocol and create standard orders for their EHR system, which made it easier on the chemotherapy nurses. According to Sprandio, this standardization of chemotherapy administration and treatment of side effects made care more consistent, thereby reducing mistakes and saving money through efficiency.

The Hoag Orthopedic Institute has standardized its pre-operative processing of patients. Initially, the motivation was to decrease surgical site infections, but this eventually also became a way of ensuring that all patients received what the surgeons and pre-op physicians collectively deemed the "best" care:

At Hoag there was a pre-admission screening, and the surgeon used to do it, but they did it however they wanted to. Haphazardly. Dr. Robinson from infection control supported standardizing it. Now, it all begins 3 weeks before the patient is admitted for surgery. They get MRSA-tested [tested for Methacillin-resistant Staphylococcus aureus, a serious drug-resistant skin infection]. If they test positive, they get decolonized according to a standard protocol. If they are still positive, the infectious disease team decolonizes them and reschedules the case.

The night before and the morning of their surgeries, all Hoag patients are instructed to wipe themselves down with Sage cloths, special wipes that kill bacteria on the skin. When they arrive at Hoag on the day of their surgery all the patients get a nasal iodine swabbing. They are also given antibiotics—the same antibiotics for all patients unless they have allergies—one hour before surgery. Next, the patients are all warmed up as they are being prepared for surgery. Antibiotics are stopped 24 hours after surgery using the same standing post-op orders for all patients. Throughout the entire surgery experience every Hoag patient is treated the same. As one of Hoag's senior physicians put it: "Each of the steps is a tiny, tiny little thing. But it is putting it all together in one standardized process that leads to consistent, high-quality care." As Hoag's annual outcomes report available on the internet shows, its surgical-site infection rate is less than half the expected rate based on its patient population. This standardization also applies to Hoag's rehabilitation care after surgery and how it manages postoperative pain.

Other organizations standardize care using a slightly different approach. Rather than reinvent the wheel and create their own standardization protocols from scratch, CareMore has adopted standardized care protocols for their major illnesses from professional societies, government agencies, or other authoritative bodies. As one senior CareMore official explains, "We tend not to develop our own care pathways. We take what is out there. For instance, we just use the American Diabetic Association's care pathway for managing insulin."

What makes CareMore distinctive in the standardization field is that it subjects these standardized protocols to what CareMore's CEO Sachin Jain calls an "affordability filter." As a Medicare Advantage plan, most of CareMore's patients are on fixed incomes. Ensuring that patients

adhere to their treatment plans requires that they are affordable. Therefore, CareMore selects medications, tests, and other interventions that
explicitly minimize costs for the patients. For instance, there are new
"designer" insulins that are modified to have different absorption characteristics that more closely approximate normal physiological insulin
secretion. But these new insulins are much more expensive and often
hard for patients to afford. Instead of using them, CareMore's standardized protocols recommend lower-cost 70:30 insulin. So far, CareMore
has converted about 70% of its diabetic patients to the lower-cost insulins. Tellingly, this led to a significant *improvement* in glucose control,
with a half-point drop in hemoglobin A1c measures across the entire
CareMore population. Why? Because at the lower price, patients could
afford to use the medication properly instead of skimping to save money.

Kaiser Permanente Mid-Atlantic also has its own standardization initiatives, which have been built into standardized order sets. This standardization of order sets relieves physicians and teams from having to
actively order and track the progress of patient tests, significantly improving efficiency. For instance, if a physician suspects that a patient
might have hepatitis C, the physician merely clicks on a standard order
set for the hepatitis C screening test and does not have to monitor results
or write any subsequent follow-up orders depending upon the results. If
the antibody screen is positive, the sample is automatically—based on
the "if ... then" conditioning in the original order and without the physician or health team ordering another test—sent for RNA-level analysis.
If that, too, is positive, the patient is then scheduled for a liver stiffness
test to assess the extent of the disease. Ultimately, the tests for a work-up
are all completed automatically, and a consultation with a gastroenter-
ologist specializing in hepatitis C is seamlessly arranged if the patient is
deemed to have the infection. All of this originates from just one order
by a physician. Kaiser Permanente ensures that all patients with hepatitis C are treated on this same standardized protocol, which is consistent
with both professional society guidelines and its own experts.

WESTMED also has standardized protocols that are built into standardized order sets for their electronic health record (EHR) system.
Unlike CareMore, WESTMED used a 4-pronged approach to implement these protocols: (1) the physicians themselves build the protocols and algorithms, (2) the treatment algorithms are integrated into

WESTMED's EHR, (3) physicians' adherence to the protocol and actual outcomes are monitored, and (4) annual financial bonuses are tied to how frequently they use the protocols.

The WESTMED physicians look at the available protocols, then agree among themselves on the best way to manage patients. Developing these treatment protocols is often part of the annual quality improvement projects that WESTMED requires each medical division to engage in. Following their creation, these physician-authored protocols then become part of the WESTMED EHR. For example, when the physician goes in to see a patient, that physician may see at the top of the EHR, in red, that blood pressure has been measured and is high. The physician is then encouraged to use the hypertension algorithm that a committee of WESTMED internal medicine physicians formulated. This ultimately ensures physician buy-in.

What does it mean for physicians to be "encouraged" to use WESTMED treatment algorithms? First, physicians are told that selecting the order set with prespecified medications and follow-up is more efficient than if they had to go through and select their own medication and monitoring schedule themselves. This is because the algorithm, with its built-in standard orders, saves them some time when they are seeing the patient. Second, WESTMED ties part of the physicians' annual bonuses to their use of the algorithm as well as to their hypertension control rates. According to Dr. Schwartz, "The result of having standardized orders is that we started off at about 77% of our hypertensive patients under good control. Now we are at 84%, which seems to be about the best we can do. That is compared to a national average of about 50%."

In the end, many physician organizations nationwide are trying to ensure that Ms. Wolf's experience with her children's differing annual exam does not become commonplace. "The annual exam is worthless, worthless," says WESTMED's CEO Dr. Schwartz:

> Everyone does it differently, and no one is sure what they are doing and why they are doing it. A 45-year-old guy comes in. You tell me: what are you doing the physical for? You're going to check his eyes, you're going to check his ears? And then you're going to order a whole bunch of routine blood tests. None of that brings any value to the patient or the health system.

Instead of a haphazard, worthless annual physical, WESTMED is migrating to performing annual visits modeled on the Medicare wellness visit. According to Dr. Schwartz, "In the next 18 months we want to transform all of our primary care physicals into structured, standardized, and age-appropriate wellness visits."

Similarly, Aledade, a company that helps manage primary care groups in ACO arrangements, already has standardized its adult wellness examination based on the Medicare wellness visit. They make sure patients are assessed for polypharmacy to determine whether they may have too many medications that might adversely interact, as well as for blood pressure, obesity, cholesterol and lipids, smoking and smoking cessation, depression and anxiety disorders, and, depending upon age, cognitive impairments and fall prevention. As an example, for a 45-year-old man, you might screen for anxiety and depression, recreational drug and alcohol use, obesity, exercise, and cardiovascular risk score. In addition, every person of the same age gets the same standardized wellness check-up, not just whatever arbitrary exams a primary care physician decides that day are appropriate based on what they are used to ordering or their last memorable patient had.

Standardization that becomes the routine has many advantages. First, it ensures that the highest level of care is systematically provided. Standardization allows care to always be consistent with professional society or government guidelines. All patients with hepatitis C, for example, get the right tests and a consultation with an expert. Or, in the case of Ms. Wolf's children, both children would have been screened for physical activity, and both would have been given the professional society's standard treatment for seasonal allergies. Second, as Toyota showed long ago, "Standardization promotes effective teamwork." Unlike the nurse at Ms. Wolf's pediatrician's office who did not know how to perform a screening eye exam, with standardized protocols that they routinely perform, staff are not improvising or trying to remember what treatment regimen each physician prefers. With standardized treatment protocols all staff know what tests and treatments are used and execute them as a matter of habit. With these habits, mistakes and errors decrease.

Third, standardization of care translates into standard order sets, like Kaiser Permanente's hepatitis C order set or WESTMED's hypertension order set, that can be automated. This ensures that patients get the right care without relying on physician or nurse vigilance that often fatigues and fails. And it ensures efficiency—once automated, the orders do not need to be recreated for each patient every time.

Finally, standardization also enables innovation and improvement. The physicians, medical assistants, and care managers can see how they perform and then improve their own standards of care. If their blood pressure control results are not optimal, they do not have to guess whether the problem is inconsistency. They can see whether the standardized order set results in better control of patients' blood pressure. If not, they can adjust a standard medication or make some other modification and assess its impact on the outcome. Furthermore, by allowing physician input into care protocols, medical organizations are able to foster progressive, incremental improvements in their quality of care.

PRACTICE 5: CHRONIC CARE COORDINATION

Ms. Rodriguez is an older patient who lives in a dusty town in the far southern tip of Texas. She is a diabetic, and for years her blood sugars were not well controlled. This led to multiple emergency room visits and hospitalizations. Within the last few years, however, her care has changed. Ms. Rodriguez is now seen at her physicians' office every 2 or 3 weeks to check on her blood sugars. When she is there, Dr. Jose Pena does a test—a rapid, 5-minute hemoglobin A1c. He shares the results with her and her daughter and explains why he is concerned and how she should eat and take her insulin differently. Before Ms. Rodriguez leaves she is scheduled to come in the following Wednesday, when the clinic hosts its weekly diabetic education session. There she will talk with a nutritionist about her diet and meet other diabetic patients. After her doctor's appointment, Ms. Rodriguez initially gets a call twice a week from Ms. Brenda Castro, Dr. Pena's care coordinator, to find out what her blood sugar values are, discuss how much insulin she should be injecting, and what she should be eating.

Ms. Rodriguez is getting the "high-touch care" that all chronically ill and high-cost, high-risk patients receive from the Donna Medical

Clinic. The clinic has 4 offices that encompass 6 physicians, 6 nurse practitioners and physician assistants, and 1 nurse practitioner who makes home visits. It is part of the Rio Grande Valley Accountable Care Organization, which is composed of 18 physicians in total. The clinic and ACO serve a very poor population, characterized by an average 6th-grade education and a large proportion of dual eligibles, namely poor elderly patients who qualify for both Medicare and Medicaid. Just under 50% of their patients have diabetes, like Ms. Rodriguez.

According to Dr. Pena, director of the Donna Medical Clinic, before joining the Rio Grande Valley ACO, most of his patients were not getting optimal care. True, he and the other physicians in the clinic were providing good care to 70% or more of the patients who came to their offices. However, even with good office care, 20% of the patients were noncompliant and had many gaps in care. More importantly, 30% of the patients never came to the office. Or they died. Or their care consisted only of showing up to the emergency room. Or they came to the office only every few years. Or who knows what happened—they were just lost to follow-up. Thus, about half of the Donna Medical Clinic patients were not getting care that Dr. Pena and his colleagues were proud of.

By joining the Medicare ACO program (see page 23), Donna Medical Clinic was able to get claims information on all their Medicare patients every 2 months. This allowed them to begin identifying all of their patients, especially those who were high utilizers and those who came to the office only haphazardly. They created lists of worrisome patients: high-cost patients, diabetics with high hemoglobin A1c's, and patients who had 2 or more emergency room visits in the previous 6 months.

They changed their team structure. With some advanced payment funds from Medicare, Donna Medical Clinic hired a chronic care coordinator in 3 of their practice sites and 2 coordinators for the main office. The chronic care coordinators are, in Dr. Pena's words, the "doctor's helper." They help establish a personal relationship with each patient and his or her family. During the first office visit the physician personally introduces the chronic care coordinator to the patient and family in order to ensure they actually meet and talk. The patient also signs a formal informed consent document that notifies them that the clinic will bill Medicare for the chronic care coordinator's services and that the coordinator will monitor their EHR and call them regularly.

The chronic care coordinator has 2 key roles. First, they must review every patient who comes to the office and create a list of what services are missing—gaps in care—or which critical laboratory or other values that are abnormal, such as high blood pressure or cholesterol. They are entrusted to close these gaps in care. For instance, a chronic care coordinator might administer a flu shot or schedule a Pap smear. Then, they flag in red any abnormal test results or laboratory values the physician needs to address. This obviates the need for physicians to hunt through the medical record for the patients' latest and previous results, and it informs and focuses the physicians' care of the patients.

Second, the care coordinators provide chronic care management. They follow 40 to 50 high-risk patients and call them at least once a week. They have standardized questions they use in these calls, such as: Are you taking your medications? Of congestive heart failure patients they ask: Are you checking your weight every 3 days? What were the last 2 weights? Of diabetic patients they ask: Are you checking your blood sugars? Are you following your diet? They also talk to the critical family caregiver—typically a daughter or daughter-in-law—to be sure they understand the patient's care plan. These weekly calls also serve an unexpected secondary, yet nevertheless critical, function: for many of Donna Medical Clinic's more elderly patients the calls are the only social interaction they have. So the chronic care coordinator is providing not only chronic care management but also a valuable psychosocial and behavioral health intervention—keeping patients engaged.

Finally, the chronic care coordinators emphasize Donna Medical Clinic's "call or come" philosophy to the patients and family. Historically, the clinic's patients had a very high use of ambulances and emergency room visits. Now the clinic—with other offices in the ACO—has a clinician available on the phone 24/7. The ACO also has a clinic open from 5 p.m. to 9 p.m. every weekday as well as on Saturday and Sunday mornings for walk-ins. Furthermore, the clinic has switched to open-access scheduling (see pages 64–67) and reserves 3 office appointments as unscheduled every weekday morning for walk-ins. They try to see every walk-in every day. They tell patients that whenever they feel sick—or, if they are diabetics, when they get a blood sugar reading of less than 90 or higher than 250—to call their physician or care coordinator or to just come to the office. Disseminating this "call or come" philosophy has dramatically reduced ambulance and emergency room use.

The Rio Grande Valley ACO also created teams for complex case management targeted at the sickest 2% to 3% of their patients. These patients are either very ill or have major psychosocial disruptions— "severe problems at home"—and, according to Dr. Pena, about half of them have been diagnosed with depression. The team consists of a physician, a social worker, a pastor, and a home health agency team member. The team meets once a week to review cases and their care plans. Interventions almost invariably include home visits and more counseling than traditional medical care.

The Donna Medical Clinic also has a home-care nurse practitioner who visits the home-bound, frail, elderly patients recently discharged from the hospital, and 50 or so nursing home patients. She will bring flu or pneumonia shots and medications to patients who cannot come into the office or pharmacy. Each patient is visited at least once a month.

Rio Grande Valley ACO's results are impressive, especially given that its population base is one that is often considered to be among the hardest to manage—poor, low-educated, non-English-speaking elderly patients. For 5 key diabetes quality measures—control of hemoglobin A1c, blood pressure control, LDL-cholesterol control, smoking cessation, and aspirin use—the ACO improved its performance from 20% total control to nearly 50%; the best practice in the ACO has nearly 80% control. The ACO is also among the top 90th percentile in the country for diabetic patients that have hemoglobin A1c below 9%. The Rio Grande Valley ACO has saved more than $10 million each year since its inception in 2012.

This is what effective chronic care management looks like. Not high technology. Not complex. Just lots and lots of personal interactions ensuring that the basics are being accomplished consistently for every high-cost, high-risk patient.

Such chronic care management is critical—indeed, it may be the single most important transformational practice—because that is where the money is. Of all the dollars spent on healthcare, only about 14% are spent on acute illnesses and emergencies—broken bones, lacerations, trauma, and the like. The vast majority of dollars, about 84%, are spent on managing chronic illnesses (see Figure 4.2, page 228). And within the chronic illness category, spending is heavily concentrated on just a few patients. Although critics are right to lament the high costs that plague our enormous healthcare system, the reality is that 1% of patients consume approximately 20% of costs, 5% consume 50% of costs, and 10% of patients consume nearly 67% of costs (see Figure 4.3, page 229). These high-cost patients have congestive heart failure, emphysema, coronary artery disease, asthma, cancer, diabetes, multiple sclerosis, and other chronic conditions. Thus, to achieve the lower cost integral to the triple aim, the healthcare system needs to do a better job of caring for patients with chronic illness like Ms. Rodriguez.

In order to transform chronic care treatment, tertiary prevention is paramount. When most people hear the word "prevention," they think of primary prevention, interventions like vaccines, colonoscopies, or mammograms, that target the healthy to prevent an illness. Still others think of secondary prevention, interventions that target those at high risk of developing a condition, like prescribing statins to patients with high cholesterol to reduce the risk of a heart attack or stroke. Undoubtedly, these types of prevention are important, but—at least for the purposes of transforming the delivery system to increase quality and reduce unnecessary costs—they pale in comparison to tertiary prevention.

Tertiary prevention focuses on people with established health problems—diabetics, patients who suffered a heart attack, those hospitalized for asthma, those with depression—and aims to prevent exacerbations and complications from developing. For example, tertiary prevention for a diabetic would focus on preventing infections, gangrene, and amputations.

The key to tertiary prevention is the kind of chronic care management delivered by the Rio Grande Valley ACO and other top-performing medical organizations such as Iora Health and CareMore. As CareMore's CEO stated "Let's face it, chronic care management is not rocket science. It is doing the basics consistently." What are those basics? In general, effective chronic care management involves a 5-step process (see Table 4.2, page 226).

First, successfully transformed medical organizations have a process to identify high-risk patients. They typically rely on staff gestalt or medical intuition backed up by simple data, such as recent hospitalizations, high ER use, more than 8 prescriptions, or high-hemoglobin A1c's. Relying on physicians' recall might bias the list to include lots of "high-hassle" rather than high-risk patients, and it will frequently miss patients, like the 30% of Dr. Pena's patients who are out of mind because they do not come in to the office. Thus, combining simple, objective data and subjective physician and nurse assessments creates the best predictors of high-cost, high-risk patients.

Second, although each organization may have different primary care team configurations, all organizations physically embed a chronic care coordinator, health coach, or person like Brenda Castro from the Donna Medical Clinic within the primary care or specialty care team. They do not outsource this to a disease-management company that uses telephonic interventions or to an insurance company's call center. This co-location allows physicians to directly and personally introduce and "hand off" the patients to the care manager. According to Clive Fields, a physician at VillageMD in Houston, "If possible, the physicians introduce the care manager to the patient and family right in the exam room to create a personal connection."

Third, physician offices or health systems prioritize efficient rooming. They entrust the chronic care coordinator or the medical assistant with closing care gaps, such as scheduling a Pap smear or giving flu shots, during rooming (see pages 67–87). They do not rely on physicians to address care gaps but instead create a system outside the physician that ensures they are addressed.

Fourth, and most importantly, organizations rely on frequent touches with the patient and the primary caregiver. In the words of Dr. Pena, "The key to managing our sick patients is frequent calls, frequent appointments, and frequent home visits." Offices and health systems that have made chronic care management work do not necessarily deploy lots of technology, such as continuous glucose monitors, continuous heart monitors, high-technology pill dispensers, and remote camera monitoring. They instead rely on human-to-human contact—and lots of it—from everyone on the healthcare team. Successful places, in short, are characterized by low-tech but high-touch care.

Fifth, transformation-oriented providers maintain relentless focus on the goals of this constant contact: to educate patients about their disease, to empower patients to routinely monitor their disease, to ensure patients take their medications, to get patients socially engaged, and to change patients' instinctive reactions from going to the emergency room to first contacting the chronic care coordinator or physician's office when something untoward occurs.

Iora Health, a for-profit primary care group with 29 sites in 9 states, is another place known for its exceptional chronic care management. At Iora it all starts with the "worry score." Traditionally a physician's attention is directed to the "squeaky wheel"—the patient who calls or comes directly into the office, complaining about something and thereby alerting the physician to his or her health issue. At Iora, however, physicians' attention is trained on patients who are sick or about to become sick, regardless of whether they are being "squeaky." This is possible because of Iora's worry score, developed to steer provider time away from the worried, but relatively healthy or stable, and toward the high-risk, chronically ill.

Iora's worry score has been through 3 iterations. Each revision has seen a simplification of the score. Initially, the worry score was from 0 to 100 and served to identify the chance a patient had of being hospitalized within the next 90 days. However, this proved to be too complicated to accurately identify high-risk patients. The second-generation worry score only ranged from 0 to 10, and even this was too complex. In generation 3, the worry score has just 4 levels: emergent, high, medium, and low worry.

The health team's gestalt determines the level. In order to assign a patient a score, the health team integrates a slew of diverse information ranging from the objective—hospitalizations, recent emergency room visits, residence in an institutional facility (e.g., nursing home), abnormal laboratory values—to the subjective—the patient did not sound well on the phone with the health coach, has not responded to a phone call, recently lost a job, or is in the midst of a divorce. Rather than using a formal algorithm, the team mentally integrates this information. Iora prefers relying on physician and nurse know-how, as it has found that health team intuition has been hard won over the years and correlates amazingly well with quantitative measures based on detailed modeling of claims data. Of course, as an added bonus, relying on physician intuition is cheaper and more efficient than implementing complex predictive modeling.

Once a patient's worry score is determined, it is prominently displayed on his or her electronic health record, where it can then guide clinicians in deciding how best to care for the patient. Low-risk patients are healthy people who generally need preventive services or, at most, acute (but not life-saving) care for an accident. These patients can be cared for with a brief, annual "check-in," which, depending on the circumstances, may not need to include an in-office physical exam, but instead can be accomplished through a text message or call. Emergent patients, meanwhile, constitute just 1% to 2% of patients who are on the "crisis board." They are hospitalized or confronting a serious crisis. The key patients, however, are those who are categorized as high risk because their trajectories can be dramatically improved by a healthcare team intervention. High-risk patients represent 8% to 9% of all Iora patients and typically have either multiple chronic conditions, some of which may be poorly controlled; social problems, such as family or housing issues; or mental health issues. These patients receive sustained attention from a health coach in order to avoid needing acute medical services.

Iora also has a slightly unique primary care team structure. Iora's chronic care coordinator equivalent is called a *health coach* who is paired with a primary care provider and works in the same office. The health coach typically follows 20 to 40 high-risk patients at a time. He or she is responsible for rooming patients during office visits, closing care gaps, talking to patients outside of office appointments about their health or any complicating psychosocial issues, and performing motivational interviewing combined with behavioral modification coaching.

At Iora Health care centers, each day begins with a 45-minute team huddle with the primary care physician, health coach, clinic manager, administrative staff, and others. The main focus of these huddles is to identify which patients are "in crisis or in trouble," review already identified emergent or high-risk patients, and map out what interventions—a call, an office visit, a home visit—should be initiated, and by which team member, for patients on the crisis board.

Yet another model of chronic care management comes out of Care-More, a Medicare Advantage plan, now owned by Anthem. CareMore is headquartered in southern California and focuses on frail elderly. Its model for its expensive, chronically ill patients is built on high-touch interactions, extending the time of care, and effectively implementing well-accepted guidelines and treatment pathways. To that extent CareMore's secret sauce for managing its chronically ill patients is, according to Dr. Sachin Jain, a Harvard-trained internist and CareMore's new CEO, actually pretty simple:

> Let's face it, our pitch deck is the same as everyone else's. We're all using the same talking points. But what we *do* is different. The roles are different. The sites of care are different. The engagement model is different. The time spent with patients is different. . . . It is funny, if we have one complaint from our patients, it is that they see and hear from CareMore staff too much.

Ultimately CareMore prioritizes *time* above all else in their patient care.

CareMore uses multiple methods to identify patients with chronic illnesses, but none involve high-tech, predictive algorithms. Their most successful approaches are relatively old fashioned: using physician intuition, recent hospital discharges, worrisome labs value, and frequency of appointments. Patients who are identified as high risk are placed on a "war board" in the clinic center, a sort of white board used to track those patients deemed high risk. As one CareMore physician explains, the war board has many benefits:

> Anyone can put a patient up there: hospitalist, care manager, medical assistant. And it is basically any patient that we think is frail or high risk. We usually put the patient's name, a little bit of their diagnosis, the last time they were admitted, and the last time we contacted them. In addition, all the "red" patients that we identify on our daily rounds—patients who we think are at high risk of hospital admission or readmission—go on the war board.

At least once a month the whole center team reviews the 25 or so patients on the "war board":

> We also have monthly meetings where we go over all those patients with the whole center team—case manager, doctors, social workers, house

call team, behavioral health. We all get together and review those cases and try to actively manage them, keep them healthy, and keep them out of the hospital.

In this way the highest-risk patients are rarely lost to the system and instead are actively tracked and discussed in order to prevent future hospitalizations.

CareMore does not directly employ their own primary care providers; rather, they contract out community physicians to care for CareMore patients. They pay the primary care providers a guaranteed monthly payment, also known as a capitation—but they don't call it that. The guarantee is the average annual payment for CareMore's Medicare patients—which is typically 6 or 7 primary care provider (PCP) visits per year, divided into 12 monthly installments.

Community PCPs are encouraged to refer patients they find difficult to care for to a CareMore physician. Local PCPs usually refer patients with uncontrolled hypertension, brittle diabetes, medication noncompliance, or those who are seeing their physicians too many times a year. Normal physician reluctance and worry that CareMore might "steal" their patients is mitigated because there is no financial penalty—physicians still get their guaranteed monthly payment. Furthermore, this frees up time on the community physicians' schedule to see other fee-paying patients.

Yet another way of identifying high-risk patients is CareMore's Healthy Start exam. Every elderly person who signs up for CareMore gets a 1-hour, comprehensive "head-to-toe examination that covers all their medications, all their past medical history, all their requirements." The Healthy Start exam also screens for mental health issues, cognitive deficits, and social situations. About 80% of new enrollees obtain a Healthy Start exam. The exam offers significant financial advantages for CareMore, as it allows the team to identify and register all comorbidities for Medicare's risk adjustment, thereby ensuring higher reimbursements right from the start. It is also cost effective, as it is performed by CareMore employed nurse practitioners rather than physicians. Most importantly, the Healthy Start exam often uncovers both acute and chronic problems, such as uncontrolled hypertension, chronic renal failure, or depression, enabling CareMore physicians to immediately intervene before an ER visit or hospitalization identifies the problem at substantial costs.

CareMore also identifies all patients who have been hospitalized. Many such patients are in for elective procedures and can receive follow-up from their local primary care physician, but others are seriously ill and need intense CareMore follow-up.

Finally, CareMore trolls its data for what might be called "red flags" such as diabetic patients who have 2 sequential high hemoglobin A1c measurements, patients who are prescribed anticoagulants, or "patients [like Miss Harris] who are 95 and seeing 6 doctors." CareMore also uses predictive modeling to determine a community assessment risk score that takes into account factors like number of hospitalizations, chronic conditions, and medications in order to identify chronically ill patients in need of additional attention.

Once these patients are identified, CareMore does not wait for patients to come to them; instead, they reach out to these chronically ill patients and pull them into the system. For instance, patients diagnosed with health issues through the Healthy Start exam do not leave until they have met with a chronic care coordinator, have scheduled appointments with a dietician or a psychotherapist, are put on the right dose of hypertension medication, are trained to use a telemedicine blood pressure cuff, or have a follow-up appointment with the nurse practitioner scheduled. Similarly, patients identified at hospital discharge have a follow-up home visit or clinic appointment arranged for them before they are discharged. Other patients are proactively contacted. As the former CEO of CareMore, Leeba Lessin, says,

> So 90% of American primary care happens because someone doesn't feel good, they wake up in the morning, they make a call. . . . But in our case there are a variety of daily, weekly, monthly activities that create outbound activities on our part that are really primary care. . . . We make an outbound call to the person who got the Coumadin script and have them come into our anticoagulation clinic and start getting their INR managed and so forth.

CareMore has built teams to care for these sicker, chronically ill patients with the intention of heaping outpatient services on them, thereby forestalling exacerbations that would require expensive emergency room visits and hospital admissions. Like Rio Grande ACO and Iora, CareMore also has its own chronic care coordinators. The CareMore care managers work side-by-side with the physicians, nurse practitioners, and other care providers. They get to know patients face-to-face rather than over the phone so that when they call a patient, there is already an existing personal relationship.

Another key team member is a unique CareMore provider: the extensivist. The extensivist expands the role of the traditional hospitalist into a more comprehensive chronic care physician. Extensivists see about 6 to 10 hospitalized CareMore patients each morning. This is a comparatively light load so as to free up time for care activities outside of the hospital and to reduce extensivist burnout. In the afternoon, the extensivists then join all the nurse practitioners and chronic care coordinators to review every single case in the hospital and identify what needs to be done to discharge the patients to a skilled nursing facility (SNF), back home, or to some other arrangement as expeditiously as possible. During these meetings patients are classified into red, yellow, and green based on their assessed risk for having a complication that requires more medical care.

The green patients are those who only need a follow-up appointment with their local physicians. On the opposite end of the spectrum, as one physician put it, are the red patients "who get a phone call from the case manager immediately the next day, if the not the same day as discharge. They are the seen in the CareMore clinic within 24 to 48 hours by the extensivist." Using the bonds with the patient and family forged during the inpatient stay, the extensivist is able to provide continuity of care in their afternoon clinics at the CareMore center. Sometimes this care only lasts until the patient is stable, at which time the patient's management is returned to their community-based primary care physician. Other times, such as for patients with end-stage congestive heart failure or emphysema, the extensivist becomes the patient's physician for the rest of their lives. Extensivists also take over the care of high-risk, chronically ill patients identified by the other mechanisms: "This model gives the extensivists ownership of that patient." About 20% of CareMore patients are cared for by the extensivists, some for a short time and others for their remaining lifetimes.

Another key part of the CareMore philosophy for chronic illness management is the creation of specialized clinics designed to manage particular problems that, if left untreated, can lead to emergency room visits, hospitalizations, and higher costs. As previously noted, CareMore has an anticoagulation clinic. This clinic is run entirely by medical assistants (MAs) rather than physicians or nurses. The MAs only perform anticoagulation education, monitoring, and medication adjustments, but they make sure they get to know each patient individually. CareMore also has a specialized clinic for diabetic foot care that cuts patients' toenails, trims corns, and cares for small cuts. CareMore uses these clinic appointments to educate patients about a variety of health issues, such as the importance of taking good care of their feet to prevent debilitating and expensive infections, gangrene, and amputations. As one senior CareMore executive explains,

> Who is the best person to prevent diabetic amputation? The patient.... At the end of the day, an individual who knows that any breach of their skin requires instant attention is the most important tool in ultimately preventing a diabetic amputation.
>
> So we think that patients who understand what's actually happening in their body are better helpers.... We tell them, "Here's why your feet are vulnerable, here's why a breach of the skin won't heal, here's why you might not feel it, here's why you need to check your feet."
>
> We think patients need to know why their feet matter long before they have a big, open, unhealed wound. And that leads us at CareMore to have services to remove their corns and trim their nails. The reason we are trimming their corns is that if they try to take their own corn out, they are going to put a hole in their foot. And we'd rather they not do that.

The CareMore foot clinic also provides a monthly opportunity for chronic care coordinators to interact with diabetic patients and see if they are using their insulin properly, eating properly, and if there are any stressors in patients' lives that might be leading to uncontrolled glucose levels.

The foot clinic is not the only program CareMore has for its diabetics. It also has a nurse practitioner spend time with each patient to explain the medications and to offer dietary assistance to help patients "understand how to read labels on the cans of food that they are buying." Recently, one pharmacist started meeting with patients who have 10 or more medications. As one physician describes the program: "She'll see patients and try to cut down on the polypharmacy and identify high-risk medications. She also helps with medication adherence, especially in the diabetic patients." In these ways healthcare providers besides physicians are able to help contribute to patients' care.

CareMore is also aware that this kind of chronic care requires constant attention. CareMore recently found that its staff was slipping. They were not enrolling all their diabetic or congestive heart failure patients in their care programs. In order to tackle this decline in care, CareMore renewed its clinical outreach efforts—reviewing abnormal labs, disease registries, and patient lists. They were ultimately able to increase the percent of eligible patients enrolled in disease programs from 20% back to 70%. Even the best, longstanding programs require constant attention.

For years many people have known that care management of patients with chronic illness is critical to delivering high-value care. Many attempts at chronic care management have failed to produce results. There are many reasons for the failure. Places that have succeeded, however, seem to all do it by following the same 5 steps (see Table 4.2, page 226). Critical to their success is physically co-locating the care managers with physicians and other clinicians, making them an integral part of the patient's care team, and initiating frequent personal contacts with the patient. This kind of care management has allowed transformed practices to reduce the costs of caring for these patients by 20% or more.

THESE 5 PRACTICES—from scheduling, registration, and rooming to performance measurement, standardization of care, and chronic care coordination—are mainly focused on transforming the physician's office. Fortunately, there is significant experience at numerous organizations on how these practices should be changed. Ultimately, these groups have all come to very similar conclusions on how best to change. For instance, scheduling should be removed from the physician's control; offices should go to open access scheduling, with 20% to 50% of appointments left open at the start of every day. Similarly, there are 5 consistent steps needed for successful chronic care coordination, with the most important being co-location of chronic care managers with physicians, forging personal relationships between managers and patients, and frequent—and I mean *really* frequent—contact with the patient. Each of the medical organizations that has transformed care does it basically the same way. What differentiates successful organizations from more retrograde ones is that they follow these steps and, more importantly, are relentless in their execution. Successful practices and health systems make sure to work out all of the large and small challenges that arise while also recognizing that change takes time (see Chapter 8).

In the next chapter we will focus on transforming relationships with other healthcare providers—the importance of introducing shared decision making for preference-sensitive conditions, especially expensive procedures; of selectively working with only high-performing specialists, hospitals, and other facilities; and of focusing on the systematic de-institutionalization of care. Because so much of the cost of care revolves around procedures, specialist care, and institutional care, these transformational practices are important in reducing unnecessary care and the per-unit cost of care delivery.

Chapter 5

THE TWELVE PRACTICES
OF TRANSFORMATION

Transforming Provider Interactions

PRACTICE 6: SHARED DECISION MAKING

Like 31 million other Americans, George, a colleague of mine, has had excruciating lower-back pain for years. It all began in his junior year of college when he helped his then-girlfriend move out of her apartment. Despite being a weightlifter and working on the grounds crew at a golf course, the move resulted in awful spasms that left him on the floor for hours. A few years later, in 2010, George was weightlifting in a hotel gym when his back gave out, causing him to drop the dumbbell and break his index finger. Following this incident George was taken to a hospital and immobilized for 2 days. MRIs from his hospitalization showed that George had a bulging disc in his lumbar spine.

In the winter of 2014, George began experiencing nerve pain. By his account he had been suffering from pneumonia and was coughing violently for several weeks. Once he recovered, George then took his 2 daughters to a "fun house," where he bounced on a trampoline with them. While bouncing he felt what he described as a "tweak" in his back. The pain soon worsened and shot down his left leg. After this incident the pain waxed and waned. On certain days it was so debilitating that George could not concentrate on his work. His primary care physician ordered an X-ray and then an MRI, which showed 2 bulging discs, one at L4-L5 and another at L5-S1. George was faced with a number of options: physical therapy, pain medication, steroid injections, or back surgery. Ultimately, George's decision was a judgment call.

Treatment for back pain is a classic "preference-sensitive" condition. Which option a patient pursues and how long they pursue that option for, depends on how they weigh the pain, the chances of pain relief with various interventions, the time it takes to get pain relief, the risks of interventions, and so on. There are hundreds of medical conditions for which there are different therapeutic options that vary tremendously in risk, benefits, time to heal, and cost. These include surgical procedures ranging from hip and knee replacements for pain caused by osteoarthritis, to breast surgery for cancer, to stents or medical treatment of chronic stable angina, to surgical or medical treatments for an enlarged prostate, and even to aspirin for the prevention of heart attacks. In the end, the patient must usually rely on instinct to make the final call. Such decisions are informed by technical medical information, but are fundamentally trade-offs between different risks, symptoms, and side effects—all over different time horizons.

For many patients like George, what intervention they get often depends on which physician they happen to see first and how these various options are—or are not—presented. According to the Commonwealth Fund, for example, less than half of adult patients facing a medical decision report that their provider ever asked them about their goals and concerns for treatment.

Within the past several decades many physicians have begun to argue that such decisions should be made with—rather than for—the patient. This approach is known as "shared decision making," a systematic process in which patients, like George, are provided with information about the medical intervention usually accompanied by some kind of formal decision aide, a document, or more frequently, video, or computer program that guides patients through the procedure, its purpose, its risks and benefits based on published data, and often patient testimonials. The patients are then allowed to make their decision based on the information they received, their preferences, and discussions with their physicians.

Studies of decision aides and shared decision making have proven their advantages along several dimensions of quality and cost. A 2014 Cochrane Collaborative review of 115 studies involving over 34,000 patients revealed encouraging results, both in terms of patients' knowledge and reduced use of expensive services. The summary states that decision aides and shared decision making:

a) improve [patients'] knowledge of the options (high-quality evidence);
b) [make patients] feel more informed and more clear about what matters most to them (high-quality evidence);
c) [allow patients to] have more accurate expectations of possible benefits and harms of their options (moderate-quality evidence); and
d) [allow patients to] participate more in decision making (moderate-quality evidence).

In some cases, such as with hip replacements, the use of decision aides also reduced the number of patients who chose high-cost tests and treatments.

Based on some of this research, section 3506 of the Affordable Care Act was created as a "sleeper provision" that was supposed to fund an independent agency to certify decision aides. For a variety of reasons, mainly the lack of enthusiastic support from the federal government, this part of the ACA has not had much traction until recently. However, many individual physician offices, clinics, and health systems have transformed their care by implementing their own versions of decision aides and shared decision making, especially for expensive, preference-sensitive conditions. This is particularly important when considering the volume and cost of certain preference-sensitive procedures. Each year there are over 700,000 knee replacements and 330,000 hip replacements performed, as well as many back procedures for pain that, together, cost tens of billions of dollars. Even modest declines in the procedure rates, possibly as a result of patients coming to realize how long it might take to recover, and grasping that there is some real chance they won't become pain-free, or not really wanting them in the first place, can constitute significant savings with clinically equivalent outcomes and ensure care is aligned with patient preferences.

Group Health Cooperative, a traditional integrated delivery system in Washington state, now part of Kaiser Permanente, may be the most enthusiastic implementer of decision aides and the shared decision-making process. In 2009, Group Health Cooperative began a quasi-experimental trial of shared decision making, using 12 preference-sensitive conditions that included breast cancer surgery, hip and knee replacements for osteoarthritis pain, and prostatectomy for benign enlarged prostate and early-stage prostate cancer. These early trials showed important findings. Initially, when specialists such as orthopedic surgeons distributed decision aides, it was hard to integrate these decision aides into routine patient flow, so a large proportion of patients did not actually get the decision aides and participate in shared decision making. By having decision aides—either a program website or a DVD with the program video—distributed by the referring primary care physicians, however, more patients participate in shared decision making. Even without optimal use, there was a resulting quality improvement. Patients who did receive the decision aide felt like they were more knowledgeable of their treatment options, were more confident in their discussions with their physician, and had greater satisfaction in their choice of therapy. Cost savings were present but inconsistent. For instance, there was a 26% decrease in hip replacement surgery after the introduction of the decision aides and shared decision making (not all were actually given these interventions) and a 38% decline in knee replacement surgery. Overall, when taking into account the alternative intervention, these declines in surgery produced a 12% to 21% decline in costs over 6 months. However, in other cases, such as hysterectomies for benign uterine conditions, there were no statistically significant declines in either surgery rates or costs. Nevertheless, the decision aides and shared decision making did not drive up costs.

Given that it improves quality while remaining revenue neutral—or even saving costs—the shared decision-making program was more widely instituted at Group Health Cooperative through a 4-step process (see Table 5.1, page 230). First, the providers were trained. Using decision aides and, more importantly, having a conversation with patients about their preferences for medical interventions, are not a set of skills people are born with. Physicians, physician assistants, and other providers need training on the use of decision aides and on having conversations about shared decision making. This includes watching—or reading—the decision aide video and learning how to elicit and explore patient preferences. Ensuring that patients have basic knowledge about alternative interventions is, by itself, not necessarily enough.

Second, Group Health Cooperative has tried to better integrate distributing the decision aide into its workflows. Group Health Cooperative uses decision aides available on the web or on DVD for patient viewing. Because most deal with surgery or specialty care, the preferred option is for the patient's primary care physician to give them access to the decision aide prior to seeing the surgeon or specialist.

Third, after completing the decision aide, patients are asked to complete a "feed-forward" questionnaire. This evaluates patients' knowledge of their options, their preferences, and which intervention they are leaning toward. This patient information is then sent to the surgeon or specialist through the Group Health Cooperative EHR in order to frame subsequent discussions with the patients.

Fourth, Group Health Cooperative tracks and reports back to physicians on a quarterly basis their rate of using decision aides and comparative utilization data on preference-sensitive conditions. Thus, orthopedic surgeons are informed of how many of their patients used the decision aide and how many knee and hip replacements for osteoarthritis pain they performed compared to their Group Health Cooperative peers.

Because decision aides and shared decision making can decrease utilization of treatments for preference-sensitive conditions, there can be some physician resistance to their use. Even though its physicians are salaried and thus do not make more money for performing more procedures, Group Health Cooperative nevertheless experienced some physician push-back. Physicians feared that if more men refused prostatectomies for benign prostatic hypertrophy and early-stage prostate cancer, then the need for urologists might decline. Similarly, if fewer patients opted for stents placed for chronic stable angina, Group Health Cooperative might not need as many interventional cardiologists. This worry is not without foundation. Although this is not of particular concern in primary care practices, as the decline in utilization would mostly be experienced in referrals, it is an issue in larger multigroup specialty practices and hospital-based systems where there tends to be surpluses of specialist physicians. To counter these worries, Group Health Cooperative encouraged providers to review the aides and share patients' response to the shared decision-making process. Once the dialogue surrounding decision aides changed to focusing on how to better educate patients and improve quality of decision making, physicians became less defensive.

For years Group Health Cooperative performed pilot projects with these decision aides. After seeing positive results, it became committed to systematically incorporating them into its practice. There now exist decision aides for approximately 250 conditions. One important goal is to expand beyond surgery and specialty care to deploy decision aides for primary care interventions such as cancer screening and aspirin use.

There are challenges to such an expansion, even at a place as committed as Group Health Cooperative. One is the need for iteration and frequent changes to integrate the decision aides and shared decision-making conversation into workflows. This is not a one-time event; it requires frequent adjustments—and different approaches in different departments. Another challenge is the decision aide market lacks competition. Although many organizations have created their own specialized decision aides for particular interventions, such as advanced-care planning and CT screening for lung cancer, there remain only 3 major commercial producers of large numbers of decision aides—Health Dialog, Healthwise, and Emmi. Consequently, using decision aides is not free. Group Health Cooperative would not provide me with a precise cost but said that systematic use of decision aides costs more than a DVD but less than $50 per patient. Compared to approximately $20,000 spent per hip replacement, this amount is small. At least at Group Health Cooperative, the savings on foregone hip and knee replacement and back surgeries have been sufficient to fund the whole decision aide and shared decision-making initiative.

CareMore's shared decision-making process is less formalized than that at Group Health Cooperative, but is consciously integrated into the care process for patients undergoing elective procedures. Initially, many CareMore patients with back pain were referred to local community groups for surgery. However, upon looking at the data, CareMore physicians realized that these community referrals were not actually helping patients with back pain. As one senior management official at CareMore explained, "There were more and more back surgeries being done, more and more hardware being put in, and yet there were still more and more failed backs." So CareMore changed its procedures. Because many of its patients are frail elderly, CareMore physicians elected to do pre-op clearances to make sure the patients are in the best possible condition for the proposed procedure. Patients who "require any kind of elective surgical procedure that requires general or spinal anesthesia must come into a CareMore clinic for a pre-op clearance." Another purpose of the pre-op visit is to ensure that the processes of informed consent and shared decision making are respected. For patients with back pain, the CareMore team explains to the patient the risks and benefits of the surgery—the chances they will experience pain relief, the amount of time it will take for rehabilitation, the chances they might end up not getting off the ventilator, and so on:

> Often times a patient just goes to the PCP, then gets sent right to the surgeon, and they get scheduled for surgery. And they never really wanted to have surgery in the first place. . . . They tell us, "I didn't want to have surgery. I just wanted to feel a little better, maybe some pain medications." But no one really takes the time to explain the risks and benefits and sit down with them. They're just shuffled from PCP to surgeon to the operating room.

CareMore did try formal decision aides and videos but saw only mixed results with their elderly population. Ultimately, they chose to do without such aides: "Instead, we come in and talked to them on an individual, a personal basis, explaining what the statistics are. That is actually key for our model of care—bonding with the patient rather than using forms and videos."

Ensuring true informed consent and shared decision making has another advantage—time. In many of these cases, especially back pain, knee pain, and other interventions done for pain relief, time itself can be a therapeutic intervention. Not only did CareMore lengthen the process by requiring the pre-op visit to be linked to the acquisition of informed consent, but it also partnered with a chiropractic college to provide chiropractic, acupuncture, and other services to their back pain patients:

> We went to the chiropractic college and said, "Can you do something to just buy time for this patient? Can you give them some chiropractic

maneuvers? Give them some acupuncture." Frankly, after a certain period of time, back pain for many patients tends to get better anyway,
without any kind of surgical intervention. We also give epidural injections, even though it has been shown in the literature that it doesn't
work, [but] it may give temporary relief, and that buys you time too.

Even if the chiropractic manipulations and acupuncture are not proven
in randomized trials, they will work for some fraction of cases. The
whole process—informed consent and chiropractic services—also
helps ensure that patients are getting the care they want and, to some
degree, reduces utilization of elective and expensive procedures.

Transformed practices introduce shared decision making for preference-sensitive conditions for 2 main reasons. First, it enhances the
patient experience by increasing patient knowledge and comfort with
their decisions. Second, at least for hip and knee surgery, it decreases
utilization because it seems to persuade many patients to postpone
or forego surgery for more conservative approaches. Nevertheless, as
Group Health Cooperative demonstrates, integrating shared decision
making into the workflow does requires effort and some adjustment.

PRACTICE 7: SITE OF SERVICE—
REFERRALS AND CENTERS OF EXCELLENCE

We just terminated a cardiology group in Orange County. We had a contract with them for cardiology services that capitated their payments. It
did not cover electrophysiology services. We looked at their use of electrophysiology services, and this one group in Orange County had billed
for more electrophysiology than CareMore used in all of Los Angeles.
They were just abusing that loophole. We don't need that, so we stopped
using them for all cardiology services.

That is Dr. Sachin Jain, CEO of CareMore, discussing how CareMore
carefully manage the specialists they use. Specialists generate a significant portion of total healthcare costs, both by charging for their personal appointments and by ordering additional tests and treatments

like electrophysiology. Even if primary care physicians are delivering high-quality low-cost care, costs and quality can still be thrown off because of the way specialists, hospitals, skilled nursing facilities, and other specialist providers are caring for their patients.

Compared to other countries, the United States has a high proportion of specialists and a low proportion of primary care physicians. Many factors have contributed to this situation. After World War II, the NIH funded the fellowship training of specialists and encouraged academic health centers to create more specialist programs. Both the military and VA gave higher rank and salaries to specialists. Most importantly, private insurers and Medicare paid more for procedures, which encouraged physicians to go into surgery and other medical specialties such as cardiology and gastroenterology with well-reimbursed procedures. Indeed, when the lifetime earnings of a specialist are 3, 5, or even 10 times higher than that of a primary care physician, it can tip the balance of career selection even if early-career physicians are not fixated on income.

This imbalance has important cost implications. As Chris Chen points out, there are community hospitals in Miami that have 70 cardiologists on staff—way too many for the number of patients served. As a consequence, these hospitals tend to do more procedures and get around rules that limit procedures. This is termed "supply-induced demand," a phenomenon of having more physicians in an area than is necessary, which in turn tends to drive up the number of procedures and interventions. Supply-induced demand is a well-established issue in medicine. Contrary to what many people assume—that more tests are always better and will not cause problems—geographical areas with physicians who order more tests do not produce better clinical outcomes and may, in fact, actually produce worse outcomes. An overabundance of specialists can exacerbate this problem. A 2004 study of Medicare patients out of Dartmouth came to the following conclusion:

> We find that states with higher Medicare spending have lower-quality care. This negative relationship may be driven by the use of intensive, costly care that crowds out the use of more effective care. One mechanism for this trade-off may be the mix of the provider workforce: States with more general practitioners use more effective care and have lower

spending, while those with more specialists have higher costs and lower quality. Improving the quality of beneficiaries' care could be accomplished with more effective use of existing dollars.

Physicians and health systems that have transformed their care are rearranging the site of service referrals for specialists, hospitals, and other types of care in 4 major ways. First, transformed practices are expanding primary care and utilizing specialists as consultants. Specialists are no longer managers of patients' routine care but instead are brought in only episodically to advise and to manage only the sickest patients. At Dean Clinic, Mark Kaufman, one of the physician executives, said,

> We want our primary care physicians to be competent and confident generalists. Most generalists can handle routine problems. We find that about 80% of the time the generalist already knows what the specialists are going to recommend. So getting a consultation does not necessarily enhance patient care. The generalist can and should be managing the patient.

A specific example was the management of sinus infections at Dean Clinic:

> It used to be that somebody would come in with a sinus infection, and the primary care doctor would immediately refer them to an ENT [ears, nose, and throat doctor] because the [PCP] did not have time to do the full workup. Now they have the time, and we don't need to refer so many patients to ENTs.

At Dean Clinic, the same was true of allergy and dermatology care. The clinic was able to change primary care responsibilities by changing how physicians were paid. Dean stopped paying primary care physicians based solely on the number of patients they saw, which incentivized volume instead of attending to all of the patient's real needs.

With generalists managing patients, specialists stick to their specialty. Cardiologists only manage patients' heart failure, severe coronary artery disease, low ejection fraction, and atrial fibrillation, not patients' diabetes, rheumatoid arthritis, or asthma. As one cardiologist at WESTMED put it, "What I like is that all I see is cardiology. I don't see my patients for diabetes or the other medical problems or scheduling their mammograms or flu shots. The system allows me to deliver great cardiology care."

For larger physician groups and health systems this invariably means "right sizing" the number of specialists—a fancy term for reducing the number of total specialists either by not replacing those who retire or laying off some specialists. For instance, CareMore employs only 9 cardiologists and 4 oncologists for its 80,000 frail elderly patients.

Second, almost all transformed practices and health systems, including smaller ones, also critically evaluate which specialists they send referrals to, a practice known as steerage or selective contracting. By doing so, they can identify high-value specialists—those specialists who deliver high-quality care instead of just ordering multiple tests, and who have reasonable prices for their services. At CareMore they use their own data on specialists, patient outcomes and the frequency of hospital admissions, test ordering, and other markers of utilization to select outside specialists. CareMore has recently begun to use external evaluators like RowdMap to help them determine the value of specialists.

This approach can be applied to many services, such as contracting for breast cancer radiation therapy. In the treatment of breast cancer, hypofractionation—a 3-week course in which each treatment involves increasingly intense radiation—is clinically equivalent in terms of survival, recurrence, and cosmetic outcomes to the traditional 7 weeks of radiation and is about one-third less expensive. Physicians and health systems looking to minimize costs and improve quality could therefore contract with radiation oncologists who primarily use hypofractionation. Additionally, they could contract with radiation oncologists who use only one dose of radiation, rather than the more common 10 or 20 doses, to treat painful bone metastases as this one dose treatment is clinically equivalent and significantly less expensive. (Because these terminally ill patients do not have to come back and forth 10 times, this also enhances patients' quality of life.)

VillageMD also tries to ensure that patients follow through on specialty consultations and that they be performed by high-value, high-quality (read: lower-cost) specialists is to create a referral office right in their practice sites. The referral specialist has a list of all the specialist physicians categorized by the insurance company network, location, accessibility, and efficiency of the clinical practice. VillageMD's referral specialist identifies the medical specialist and, when needed, will help the patient schedule an appointment. This increases follow-through of the specific physician recommended by VillageMD. Although patient uptake of the service is about 70%, it is especially appreciated by vulnerable patients, the elderly, the disabled, and those who have low health literacy. Concentrating referrals on a small number of specialists improves communication and coordination of care between VillageMD primary care physicians and the specific, efficient specialists—producing better clinical outcomes.

Third, larger transformed practices or health systems have set up internal centers of excellence. Rather than have multiple offices delivering orthopedic or oncology care, they are centralizing those services into a few offices and sending all their patients to them. One example is Dean Clinic in Wisconsin, which now covers 22 counties in southern Wisconsin:

> We are going through the process of matching the appropriate capacity of the healthcare system with demand. It is like the hub-and-spoke model. We are doing our own strategic planning, asking, "What do we want to do and where?" And we are going to regionalize the provision of specialty care services like orthopedics, oncology, vascular surgery, and urology. That way we don't unnecessarily duplicate high fixed costs, ancillary services, and personnel. This will reduce per-unit fixed costs per patient procedure and improve efficiency.

This process not only improves efficiency and lowers costs, but also enhances quality in 2 ways: it makes it easier to standardize care, and, in certain types of services like surgery, higher volumes are correlated with better outcomes.

Finally, transformed practices also critically examine which services should be referred out to other facilities and which hospitals they should utilize. Again, the emphasis is on using high-quality and lower-cost facilities. For instance, Hoag Orthopedic Institute went through a process to ensure its patients were going to high-value facilities after hip and knee replacement surgery.

> One of the ways we actually tried to optimize outcomes is by looking at the skilled nursing facilities and nursing homes that all of our patients were discharged to. There were about 10 or 12 different facilities. And we looked at the readmission rates by skilled nursing facility and nursing homes, and we found dramatic variation. We had 3 or 4 that did well and the rest did not. And so now we actually selectively choose to use the skilled nursing facilities and nursing homes that seem to be taking better care of our patients.

In the Alternative Quality Contracts developed by Blue Cross Blue Shield of Massachusetts, practices are held financially accountable for the total cost of care. Each month the insurer provides practices a full claims file on all their patients. That file reveals to physicians the actual payments to all other providers—specialists, hospitals, other facilities, imaging centers, and laboratories. According to Dana Gelb Safran, of Blue Cross Blue Shield of Massachusetts, "When physicians are asked to be accountable for cost, they must have pricing data available to enable them to manage those costs and help make informed referral decision for their patients." The result of this transparency on provider pricing information is that physicians and medical organizations quickly began to change referral patterns to those specialists and hospitals providing high-quality but lower-cost services. Importantly, this shift was made in ways that avoided disrupting existing clinical relationships between patients and specialists. In the early years, providers tended to first move to lower-cost settings for things like lab testing, radiology services, and routine, one-time procedures such as colonoscopies.

Later in their contracts, many providers began to make more significant referral shifts, including some well-publicized moves of referral relationships from higher- to lower-cost hospitals and specialists. For instance, Atrius Health, the current incarnation of Harvard Pilgrim and then Harvard Vanguard's medical group, initiated a more radical response to this transparency on pricing data: they changed their hospital affiliation. For decades, Atrius had admitted patients to the Brigham and Women's Hospital, a Harvard-affiliated teaching hospital in Boston. But when Harvard-affiliated Beth Israel–Deaconess Hospital, a few blocks away from Brigham, came to them with lower cost data and pledges of closer coordination to limit admissions, unnecessary tests, and procedures, Atrius switched hospitals. Overall, shifting to lower-cost sites of care produced the majority of savings in the AQC program. As published research on the Alternative Quality Contracts showed, in the first 4 years of the program "approximately 40% of the claims savings were explained by decreases in volume [or utilization of unnecessary services], with the remainder (60%) due to lower prices."

In cases where specialty services are too expensive to buy from consultants or specialty facilities, some groups have in-sourced them, even when such changes come at a high initial investment. WESTMED, for example, has done something that many would consider totally ridiculous: they spent millions on a PET-CT scanner, including over $600,000 for the lead shielding alone. Why? Outside hospitals were charging $4,000 to $5,000 for each PET-CT scan. By having their own scanner, WESTMED was able to reduce the charge per scan to just $2,000. Yet the machine sits idle for many hours a day, and Dr. Schwartz, CEO of WESTMED, likes it that way: "I don't want anybody to use the PET scanner. I like when it's empty." Because, as he says, "I'm doing 10 to 12 scans a week and will break even on the scanner with just over 600 or so scans. Then it will pay for itself." Having a lower per-unit cost than neighboring hospitals can improve value for WESTMED.

Similarly, Dean Clinic has also examined their referrals to tertiary centers to determine what services their own physicians could actually provide—reducing referrals outside the system—and which facilities provide the best care. Dean Clinic traditionally sent many seriously ill patients to the University of Wisconsin health system. But the university is an academic medical center and very expensive. There are some medical interventions that Dean will always send to the university because the number of cases are too few and the management is too complex to be replicated by Dean, such as care for burn victims or solid organ transplantation—"quarternary care that we don't do and are fine giving to the University of Wisconsin." But there are other services that do not need to go to the university. For instance, although it still refers patients with rarer cardiac conditions such as hypertrophic cardiomyopathies to the university for care, Dean is in-sourcing care for more common cardiac conditions such as atrial fibrillation. As the Dean Clinic CEO put it,

> Right now we pay $60 to $80 million out of network to the University of Wisconsin for services. . . . But there are a lot of things being sent to the university that we could take care of within Dean. Our big focus right now is leakage—that is, care out of the Dean network that we can do at high quality internally.

A main part of the motivation for examining these referral patterns is certainly cost, but quality is also a factor. By sending patients to another nonaffiliated hospital, Dean is losing the coordination of care and introducing another transition of care. It has been well documented that transitions of care are points of friction where mistakes in medications and follow-up care frequently occur.

Dean Clinic is also trying to create competition for services that it must refer to the university or similar facilities. Rather than assume all complex pediatric cases will go to the University of Wisconsin, they have explored contracts with the Children's Hospital 90 miles away in Milwaukee. This allows them to negotiate better unit pricing. As a senior management official at Dean put it, "We are trying to pit Milwaukee Children's versus University of Wisconsin for high-end tertiary and quarternary care in the hopes of lower pricing and [better] outcomes."

Maybe the best rationale for focusing on site of service and referrals comes from the experience of Aledade, a management company that partners with practices to transform care. The practices include 500 physicians in the MSSP ACO program with about 120,000 Medicare beneficiaries and some commercial ACO contracts (see pages 54–55, 92). According to Farzad Mostashari, its CEO, Aledade offers practices "data analytics and user-friendly technology to promote seamless care . . . [as well as] best practices shared by a national network of doctors, and face-to-face practice transformation support." The initial tier of transformations that Aledade has its independent primary care practices institute include scheduling changes for same-day appointments, closing care gaps related to prevention, managing care to reduce hospitalizations, and transitioning care to reduce readmissions. Interestingly, site of service was not one of the top items that the company had its primary care ACOs initially focus on.

In just 18 months, the practices improved their quality of care, encompassed an increase in wellness visits, which included depression screening, pneumonia vaccinations, hemoglobin A1c control for diabetics, and the measurement of other important outcomes. Impressively, the ACO "was in the 98th percentile of quality scores across all 327 Medicare ACOs that began in 2012 to 2014." In addition, emergency department visits, hospitalizations, and readmissions all dropped an average of between 4% to 9%. Costs for laboratory and imaging services declined. The Aledade physicians seemed to be effectively transitioning to delivering high-value care. Yet the Aledade physicians did not receive any Medicare shared savings. A fundamental reason for this was a 13% increase in hospital outpatient and facility costs. This increase was the result of 2 factors. First, many of the specialists the Aledade physicians used now worked for hospitals, and the payments they received were higher just because they were now affiliated with a hospital. This increase in fees, without a significant change in the services provided, overwhelmed the higher-value care the primary care physicians delivered. As Farzad Mostashari, Aledade's CEO, wrote,

> [Primary care physicians] must pay particular attention to specialist practices that have been bought and reclassified as hospital outpatient settings with facility fees that can double the cost to Medicare (and patients) of procedures and visits to specialists. These trends have resulted in a 5% increase in hospital outpatient costs nationwide.

Second, hospitals were upcoding to secure higher reimbursement. Upcoding is the practice of making patients' bills higher by classifying them as sicker without any change in the actual intensity of care. For instance, patients who previously were diagnosed with pneumonia were now classified as having sepsis with no bloodstream bacteria found because that diagnosis is paid at a higher level. Upcoding is being increasingly adopted by markets nationwide. [Because of upcoding, our ACO] reduced hospitalization by 2%, but hospital costs actually increased by 4%.

To address these problems Aledade is now "creating tiers of specialists and launching an affiliates program for engagement and inclusion of high-value specialists." In other words, they are taking site of service seriously and focusing their referrals on high-value specialists.

Site of service matters and can make the difference between lowering costs and sharing in savings—or not. Moving more care inside the practice or health system and steering patients to high-value clinicians, hospitals, and other facilities is fundamental to lowering per-unit costs and reducing the total cost of care.

PRACTICE 8: DE-INSTITUTIONALIZATION OF CARE

In the 1990s there was substantial concern about managed care leading to shortened hospital stays. The media condemned the 24-hour "drive through" deliveries. Commentators damned "treat-and-street" approaches that prematurely discharged sick patients. These concerns were part of what fueled the backlash against managed care at the end of the 1990s.

The culture of care has since changed. Admission to the hospital and longer inpatient stays have ceased being seen as desirable and a sign of good care, and have instead become more of a liability. One of the catalysts of that change was the 1999 Institute of Medicine report "To Err Is Human," which showed that nearly 100,000 Americans die each year from preventable medical injuries. Avoiding admissions and minimizing hospital stays became a way to avoid hospital-acquired adverse events such as infections, bed sores, and thromboemboli, which are blood clots from lying in bed too long. Additionally, research demonstrated that it was possible to treat patients at home who typically would have been hospitalized with equivalent, or even better, outcomes and faster recoveries. Other studies found a wide variation in post-hospital care, and that patients treated in skilled nursing facilities or other inpatient rehabilitation facilities often had worse outcomes. Avoiding institutionalized medical care became not only possible but also medically advisable.

Not only was de-institutionalized care frequently of higher quality, it often saved money. For many conditions, avoiding the hospital could save approximately 20% of the cost of care. Therefore, unlike the mentality of the late 1990s and early 2000s, today's mantra is de-institutionalization—moving care out of the 4 walls of hospitals, skilled nursing facilities, and other healthcare institutions. This is why I and others have predicted that many hospitals will close over the next few years.

CareMore has acted aggressively with regards to de-institutionalization, reducing admissions, and, when admissions do occur, moving patients out of the hospital as quickly as possible. On the summer day in 2016 when I visited a CareMore facility in Los Angeles, only 211 patients were hospitalized out of CareMore's 80,000 elderly Medicare patient population. Their average length of stay (LOS) was 3.7 days, compared to Medicare's national average of 5.4 days. CareMore's bed days—a measure of both hospitalization rates and length of stay—was about 960 per 1,000 members. This value is much lower than the Medicare average of over 1,700 per 1,000 members and is significantly lower than the value of the 11 worst-performing states, which have over 2,000 bed days per 1,000 members. Even in California—usually a star player on such measures—the rate is nearly 1,300 bed days per 1,000 Medicare beneficiaries. CareMore has 26% fewer bed days than its peers in California. CareMore's 30-day, all-cause readmission rate—that is, the proportion of patients who are discharged from the hospital and readmitted within 30 days—is also impressive, at 40% below the national average. A great achievement of the ACA has been the reduction of the 30-day readmission rate among Medicare beneficiaries from 19.6% to 17.5%. It is important to note that CareMore's impressively low numbers are not the consequence of having selected a healthier Medicare population. Indeed, CareMore actually cares for the frail elderly; it has a population with an average risk of 1.08—higher than the Medicare average of 1.0.

How can these types of results be achieved? All transformed practices and health systems striving for de-institutionalization of care do so via 4 strategies: (1) reduce hospitalizations, mainly by better tertiary prevention, thereby keeping patients out of the hospital in the first place (see pages 97, 224); (2) replace hospital stays with care at home; (3) reduce the length of hospital stays by quickly transitioning patients to lower-cost facilities or home care when appropriate; and (4) reduce readmissions with better transitions of care after hospitalizations. Larger physician groups and health systems can adopt all 4 approaches, while smaller physician practices typically focus on preventing hospitalizations and reducing readmissions.

Many practices and health systems work hard to prevent the need for hospitalizations in the first place. One consequence of CareMore's toe-nail clipping service for diabetic patients is to reduce the development of foot infections, gangrene, and the need for amputations, thereby preempting hospitalizations and surgical procedures (pages 105, 226). Dr. Schwartz boasts that his WESTMED obstetricians are the highest paid per delivery among all of Cigna's networks. They are highly paid not because they are better negotiators—although that may also be true—but because they reduce hospitalization and intensive care unit rates for infants. As he says,

> The costs of obstetrics is all in the number of neonatal intensive care unit days for infants. At WESTMED we have low numbers of days because we manage pregnancy well. We see women 8 weeks after their last menstrual period. We ensure good prenatal care. And we work hard to avoid any deliveries before 39 weeks. The result is very low NICU days per 1,000 deliveries.

Main Line Oncology outside of Philadelphia created a nurse-operated call line so patients experiencing side effects of chemotherapy or any other symptoms could call. The nurses follow NCI standardized protocols for managing common symptoms such as nausea and vomiting, diarrhea, mouth sores, pain, and insomnia. The practice encourages its oncology patients to call early in the day so if they need to be seen, they can come to the office rather than go to the emergency room, where there is a higher likelihood of hospital admission. This is reminiscent of the Rio Grande Valley ACO's "call or come" approach with its patients (pages 95–96). In this way, better care management of patients with chronic illness can reduce the need for hospitalizations and facilitate de-institutionalization.

The second way to achieve de-institutionalization is to substitute home care for hospital stays. Studies at the Philadelphia VA and the

Presbyterian Healthcare Services in Albuquerque, New Mexico, have treated patients with pneumonia, urinary infections, congestive heart failure, and emphysema exacerbations at home rather than in the hospital. Through randomized trials they have shown that care at home produced fewer tests, fewer falls, higher adherence to guidelines, similar readmission rates, and faster recoveries. Impressively, the program saved nearly 20% of the costs of hospitalizations.

Caring for patients who would have otherwise been hospitalized requires complex choreography. When patients call or present to the emergency room, someone has to direct them home and preempt the admission, often over the objection of the emergency room physician and hospital. They also have to coordinate the home health services and any durable medical equipment to be promptly brought to the house as well as ensure that the visiting nurse or home health agency comes and provides the appropriate treatments. This all requires cultivating good working relationships with the home health agencies and durable medical equipment contractors. Care managers frequently assume this coordination role. While this constitutes significant work, it is nevertheless a good way to provide quality care at home to many chronically ill patients.

Third, many physician offices and systems that do not own hospitals work to reduce length of stay. The key to reducing length of stay is having the physician office or system employ its own hospitalists and hospital-based care teams rather than relying on those employed by the hospital itself. In the Mid-Atlantic region, Kaiser Permanente does not own any hospitals. Instead, it selectively contracts with a few hospitals and tries to have Kaiser Permanente Mid-Atlantic actually operate parts of the hospital. As Dr. Loftus explains,

> We have worked out with our core hospitals a dedicated section or floor for our general medical and surgical patients [has] the blue Kaiser logo. Those areas are staffed by our hospitalists, our surgeons, for the most part our anesthesiologists, and for the most part our labor and delivery doctors.
>
> One reason we have our own hospitalists is to prevent the hospital doctors from ordering a lot of unnecessary tests. Another is that this improves the coordination of care with the patient's personal doctor.

Not only does Kaiser Permanente have its own physicians in the hospitals, but it also structures the team and shifts to ensure continuity of care and efficient transitions of care. Each hospitalist works for 7 days, then is off for 7 days because Kaiser Permanente "wants the same doctor to handle the patient from admission through discharge to reduce handoffs and improve care." In addition to their own hospitalists, Kaiser Permanente teams include their own "patient care coordinators physically located in the hospitals to help with discharge planning." Each coordinator is paired up with a specific physician, and together, they manage only about 15 patients. That way they can round and huddle twice a day, get to know their patients, and be efficient about discharges.

CareMore also employs its own hospitalists—the extensivists—to manage CareMore patients both in the hospital and when they transition out (see pages 56–57). One important thing the extensivists do is prevent the hospital-based physicians from ordering too many tests and treatments. Hospital-employed physicians have incentives to add unnecessary procedures and interventions solely to increase their own revenues. For example, a patient who falls at home, like Miss Harris (see Chapter 1), might get an MRI scan of the head, a cardiac catheterization, pacemaker placement, and other interventions that are highly reimbursed. More importantly, immediately upon admission the CareMore extensivist—along with the care team, which includes a case manager and nurse practitioner (NP)—begin planning for discharge and how best to transition the patient either to a skilled nursing facility or back home with home care.

CareMore applies the same techniques it uses in the hospital to skilled nursing facilities and other institutional care sites. CareMore uses skilled nursing facilities more frequently than other health systems; indeed, it actually has a higher bed day rate at skilled nursing facilities than the Medicare average. CareMore favors the use of skilled nursing facilities because they are cheaper than hospitals and, for non-ICU care, can often provide similar levels of service. However, to ensure that the care is high quality and still appropriate, CareMore extensivists actually care for their patients in the facilities. Not only does this ensure that patients get optimal care, but it also reduces readmissions to the hospital and thwarts the common gaming technique used by skilled nursing facilities of keeping patients up to the limit of days for Medicare reimbursement. By staffing its patients with its own extensivists, CareMore has eliminated the financial incentives that often motivate behaviors at skilled nursing facilities.

When patients are preparing to go home, CareMore also works closely with medical equipment vendors and home healthcare agencies to ensure that the appropriate equipment is installed before—not 3 days after—the patient arrives home. By doing so, the right care is ready for patients the moment they arrive home. Additionally, after discharge the extensivist, nurse practitioner, or other team member will frequently visit the patient at home or see them at a CareMore center in order to ensure they are healing appropriately. Seeing patients promptly after discharge from facilities has been shown to reduce readmission rates.

Why does this model work? CareMore extensivists, nurse practitioners, and care managers are not perceived as the "1-800-Just-Say-No" team, which is patients' view of so many telephonic case managers from insurance companies. High-touch care before and during a hospital say—namely, frequent visits to the patient while in care centers, regular calls with the patient, seeing the patient the moment they are hospitalized—helps foster strong relationships between the caregiver, the patient, and the patient's family. The CareMore team strives to show that they care about their patients' well-being. Consequently, their aggressive movement of the patient out of the hospital, then out of the skilled nursing facility and into the home, is not viewed as a denial of services for cost savings but rather as in the patient's best interest.

The model also works financially. CareMore, like WESTMED and Kaiser Permanente Mid-Atlantic, negotiates per diem rates rather than using a fixed DRG—the fixed payment linked to a patient's specific diagnosis that is based on Medicare's fee—with the hospitals. This generates savings on shorter than average hospital lengths of stay. Additionally, CareMore incentivizes the extensivists by tying their pay to utilization. Experienced extensivists at CareMore can earn up to a 60% bonus of their base pay depending on their levels of clinical performance and utilization. The key measures of utilization are the number of admissions per 1,000 patients, the length of stay, and readmission rates. Thus, extensivists have an incentive to prevent patients from being hospitalized and, if hospitalized, to discharge these patients quickly. Importantly, incentivizing low readmission rates ensures that extensivists are not skimping on quality of care.

The fourth method for de-institutionalization is to reduce readmission rates. The penalties in the ACA for high readmission rates have led to a national decline in readmissions from roughly 19.5% to 17.5%. But physician practices and health systems that focus on transitions of care can do much better. One of Aledade's 3 top initiatives was optimizing transitions of care. Aledade works with smaller physician offices who tend not to employ their own hospitalists. They encourage their physicians to contact the patient within 24 to 48 hours after discharge from the hospital to ask them, "How are you feeling?" If the answer is a version of "not well," a triage nurse is called in. If they are doing well, then they arrange for the patient to come to the physician's office within 7 to 14 days. The first post-hospitalization visit focuses on medication reconciliation and efforts to reduce polypharmacy to ensure the patient is taking the right medications and is educated about their disease. As they reported in a recent publication, Aledade practices "saw a decrease in 30-day all cause readmission of between 13% and 15% when compared with national benchmarks."

Aledade is a good example of a group that implemented most of these de-institutionalization practices, especially care management, to reduce initial hospitalization and efforts to reduce readmissions. Over the first year its physicians reduced hospital use by between 2% to 9%. That is the beginning of a broader de-institutionalization transformational practice.

IN CHAPTER 4, I delineated one aspect of the transformation of the delivery system—changing the practices in the physician office. In this chapter, I illustrated the importance of changing relationships among healthcare providers, changing to whom patients are referred, and changing how to handle admissions to hospitals and other facilities to ensure high-value care. In the next chapter, I explore the changes in areas that have not traditionally been considered core to patient care. These are areas that physicians and other providers have largely ignored in their processes of transformation. These undervalued fields include behavioral health, palliative care, community interventions for patients with few social supports, and lifestyle interventions. Increasingly, these areas will become more central to delivering high-value care. Incorporating more of these services into routine care will enhance the patient experience. Care will be transformed to treat the whole patient, not just the presenting physical ailments.

Chapter 6

THE TWELVE PRACTICES
OF TRANSFORMATION

Expanding the Scope of Care

THESE FIRST 8 PRACTICES occur within a practice or healthcare system. They are the ways in which physician practices, multispecialty groups, and health systems change their processes related to interacting with patients to improve quality and the patient experience while also lowering the cost of care. These are changes that need to happen within the practices and groups. Changing the scheduling and rooming practices, co-locating and embedding care managers in the care team, and changing referral patterns cannot be done effectively if they are outsourced; indeed, it makes no sense to outsource the rooming of patients, and attempts to outsource chronic care management have largely been a failure. Conversely, the next 4 practices do not have to be delivered by a patient's care team but instead can be outsourced to companies or specific providers outside the patients' main medical team. For instance, some of the best palliative care interventions are performed by companies that contract with care providers to send a palliative care nurse to patients' homes. Lifestyle changes can also be delivered by contracted gyms or other such companies. Of course, larger providers, such as a large multispecialty group or a Kaiser Permanente, might choose to integrate these services into their offerings. But these are services that can be contracted out by primary care or specialty care physicians who provide the predominant healthcare for a patient. In this sense, the final 4 transformational practices are part of the healthcare ecosystem but not necessarily part of the very fabric or infrastructure of a physician office or multispecialty group.

PRACTICE 9: BEHAVIORAL HEALTH INTERVENTIONS

Ms. Crawford is a 65-year-old woman with multiple chronic conditions: high blood pressure, emphysema, high cholesterol, osteoarthritis, and gastric reflux. Whenever her heart starts racing and she gets a "funny feeling" in her chest accompanied by nausea, she rushes to the emergency room. Last year she visited 9 times. Each time is always the same: the emergency room staff find no changes on her EKG and no indication that she is having a heart attack or any other objective medical problem such as gastric reflux or pericarditis.

Recently Ms. Crawford's primary care physician's practice did something different: they began having Dr. Randolph, a behavioral health provider, work right in their office. Ms. Crawford's physician introduced her to Dr. Randolph. She had 6 psychotherapy sessions and was started on a non-habit-forming anti-anxiety medication. The psychotherapy sessions focused on identifying the types of stressors that caused Ms. Crawford's anxiety and how she could better cope with them. Dr. Randolph and Ms. Crawford's primary care physician write notes in the same electronic health record (EHR) and have ongoing interdisciplinary communication about Ms. Crawford's case. Dr. Randolph's work—as recorded in the EHR—is reviewed by a psychiatrist who is employed by Advocate Medical Group, which is part of the Advocate healthcare system that cares for Ms. Crawford. The psychiatrist can give advice on the diagnosis and management of patients through the EHR. For patients who have diagnostic uncertainty or difficulty managing issues, there is the opportunity for the psychiatrist to conduct a diagnostic assessment through telemedicine, in which the patient is evaluated over a video link at his or her primary care provider's office.

At Advocate, located in metropolitan Chicago, behavioral health specialists like Dr. Randolph are not just co-located in the PCP's office; they are integrated into the actual care of patients like Ms. Crawford. By co-locating behavioral health providers in the same facility, the level and quality of behavioral health services are enhanced. Moreover, cultural barriers to receiving care are reduced. Most importantly, communication between behavioral health providers, primary care physicians, and specialist physicians is greatly improved. Currently, Advocate has 13 providers co-located in 8 primary care practices in the Chicago area.

This type of practice is dubbed the collaborative care model, which was originally developed at the University of Washington in Seattle. The model employs evidence-based medications and psychosocial treatments for goal focused therapy, with goals such as reducing re-admissions from depression or, in Ms. Crawford's case, emergency room visits due to anxiety. Embedded behavioral health clinicians assist primary care providers through regular consultations and treatment adjustments for patients who may not be improving. Advocate has tweaked the original collaborative care model to keep its therapeutic intent while making it work practically within Advocate's clinical practice settings. The behavioral health specialist and the primary care physician share the same EHR and can see each other's notes and medication orders. In addition, the PCP personally hands off the patient to the behavioral health specialist, discussing the case with the specialist and introducing the specialist to the patient. Further, the behavioral health specialist and PCP work for the same organization, so their quality and cost incentives are aligned.

This is not the only behavioral health innovation Advocate is trying. It also is shifting toward a more proactive model for identifying patient with unrecognized behavioral health conditions to facilitate earlier care and treatment. For instance, Advocate has instituted systematic behavioral health screening for hospital patients who are 65 years and older and are in the emergency room or on the medical or surgical floors. Patients are screened for depression (using the Patient Health Questionnaire-9, or PHQ-9) and anxiety (using the Generalized Anxiety Disorder-7, or GAD-7). Patients who screen positive are seen by a psychiatrist, psychologist, licensed clinical social worker, or behavioral health nurse practitioner within 24 hours. It is even faster for more acute patients. At several Advocate hospitals, these consultations are performed via telehealth to provide access to psychiatrists who are in short supply. Interestingly, with this inpatient consultation in place, the Advocate hospitalists and nurses are now referring other patients who are not necessarily screened, but have other behavioral health conditions such as substance abuse, or who did not test positive on the screening questionnaires but the hospitalists and nurses think would still benefit from a behavioral health intervention. The senior executives at Advocate consider these types of behavioral health specialists as "mission critical," especially for patients for whom they assume full financial risk.

Why does Advocate consider behavioral health mission critical? The short answer is that it improved their health outcomes and financial situation. Behavioral health issues can be broadly divided into 2 categories. The first are patients whose primary diagnosis is a serious mental health disorder—schizophrenia or bipolar disorder. These are patients with complex problems who are often disabled by their illness, need to be managed by psychiatrists, and might need long- or short-term inpatient care. But there is a much broader group of patients, like Ms. Crawford, for whom behavioral health issues accompany underlying physical health problems. To use healthcare jargon, these patients have comorbid behavioral health conditions. Advocate found that behavioral health comorbidites like depression and anxiety were common, occurring in 26% of their hospitalized patients. This is consistent with national studies that have found that approximately 30% of medical outpatients and patients admitted to acute general hospitals have behavioral health comorbidities.

These behavioral health comorbidities cause suffering and are debilitating in and of themselves. But they frequently exacerbate the underlying chronic illnesses, making patients more challenging to manage and driving up healthcare costs. For example, although diabetic patients are more expensive than average patients, those who also have nonserious mental health issues are even more expensive, and those with serious and persistent mental health issues—that is, those with functional impairments that substantially interfere with life activities, such as hygiene or employment—are the most expensive (see Figure 4.2, page 228). The same is true for congestive heart failure and emphysema. As any experienced nurse or physician will tell you, when a patient with previously well-controlled diabetes or congestive heart failure starts having health problems—such as their sugars go out of whack, they suddenly gain 6 pounds of fluid, or they turn up at the emergency room with difficulty breathing—more often than not it is because some behavioral health problem has arisen. In these cases a patient like Ms. Crawford usually has become anxious about something else in their life, something that has made her upset or fretful. As a result, she might stop taking her medications properly, eat foods she shouldn't be eating, and stop doing her daily walks. Next thing you know, the Ms. Crawford–type of patient is having an expensive rendezvous with the medical system.

For decades, mainly driven by stigma and high payments, behavioral health was siloed and segregated from primary and specialty care clinicians. Behavioral health providers were relegated to different locations from primary care physicians, used different medical records, and were basically not in communication with the rest of the healthcare system.

This siloed approach is now changing. Most transformed practices and systems are well on their way to effective care management of patients with chronic illness (see Chapter 4, pages 93–106). They are improving quality and squeezing costs out of the system. At some point, they will be performing chronic care management so well that there will be few additional quality and cost gains to be achieved just with excellent care management of chronic illnesses. This is when tackling behavioral health problems comes in. To secure additional quality improvement and cost savings, transformed practices like Advocate are trying new approaches to behavioral health, especially ones focused on patients with comorbid depression and anxiety disorders. Almost all these efforts are in the early stages. They might best be thought of as mini-experiments. For instance, at Advocate, which has 6,300 employed and aligned physicians, the integrated PCP-behavioral health collaborative care model that treated Ms. Crawford has been implemented in only a few of the larger practices. The Advocate leadership expects to expand this model to additional sites in the coming year.

Advocate is not unique. No one seems to have "solved" the problem of how best to address behavioral healthcare issues for their patients. Hence, there are a variety of yet to be fully proven approaches. But many are nonetheless promising. At Advocate, they found that inpatient screening and behavioral specialist treatment decreased the direct cost for patients receiving behavioral health interventions. Interestingly, the cost of treating some chronic medical conditions for those with comorbid behavioral health problems also decreased compared to costs for managing those patients who had no behavioral health comorbidity. The magnitude of cost reductions was unanticipated, prompting Advocate leadership to promote additional investment in the delivery of behavioral health services and the integrated care.

There are other behavioral health experiments of note even at smaller physician practices. Mike Nagoshi is head of Hawaii's Central Medical Clinic, a 16-physician practice that includes 9 internists, 3 pediatricians, 2 surgeons, and 2 obstetricians. He describes a young woman who recently was in his office:

> This woman had postpartum depression and was suicidal. Uncertain what to do, her family brought her in. She insisted she would not see a psychiatrist. At the end of our appointment I asked her to accompany me down the hall. I then introduced her to the health psychologist who works in our office space. He began seeing her right then.
>
> This is a warm hand-off that we never had before. We used to refer patients to psychiatrists, but most never made it either because they did not make the appointment or it was so far into the future that they forgot. Now the psychologists are co-located in our offices, and we literally share the patients. There is no gap when I want a patient to see the psychologist.
>
> The family said it was the most remarkable intervention. It saved her life.

Two and a half years ago Dr. Nagoshi and his partners were in the midst of transforming their practice. With help of their main payer, Hawaii Medical Services Association (HMSA)—the Hawaii Blues plan—they added a care manager and dietician to their primary care teams. Then they invited a group of health psychologists to share their office space. Initially it was for 2 half-days per week; now the psychologists are in-office up to 4 full days per week. The psychologists remain independent practitioners. They bill separately from Dr. Nagoshi's Central Medical Clinic. Just recently the psychologists began putting their notes in the clinic's EHR so they can see the medical notes and the clinic's physicians can see the behavioral health notes.

From Dr. Nagoshi's perspective, there are several major advantages of co-location and shared management of patients with behavioral health problems. The physicians at Central Medical Clinic always were urged to screen for depression, anxiety, and other behavioral health conditions, but they had no effective way of getting patients who tested positive actual behavioral healthcare. As Dr. Nagoshi puts it, "Screen and refer never worked. Co-location with warm hand-offs works. Patients—even ones, like this woman, who are resistant to behavioral health providers—get care." Initially the physicians only referred patients who screened positive for depression and anxiety. With more experience—and education by the psychologists—Central Medical Clinic's primary care physicians are now referring patients for stress management, sleeping problems, and smoking cessation. Most surprising to Dr. Nagoshi is that the psychologists have been able to help with noncompliant patients, ones who used to be so frustrating for the clinic's physicians.

One unexpected advantage of having the psychologists—along with chronic care managers and other team members—practice with the primary care physicians is making it easier to recruit physicians. According to Dr. Nagoshi, "The new crop of physicians see the infrastructure—our EHR, performance reports, and especially these new team members—as helping to take some of their work. They augment the work doctors can do."

But Dr. Nagoshi recognizes that this is a work in progress: "We still don't know how to fully integrate the psychologist into our practice." He thinks the separate billing means that the clinic and the psychologists' practice are not yet seamlessly integrated. Dr. Nagoshi cannot refer every patient he wants to the psychologists because some might have a separate copay or the psychologist is not in the patient's network.

CareMore offers another experiment with integrating behavioral health into a transformed health system. During the new CareMore enrollee's 1-hour Healthy Start exam with a nurse practitioner (see page 102), services include screening tests for depression, anxiety, cognitive deficits, and other behavioral health conditions. In addition, CareMore has incorporated an annual depression screen into its treatment pathways and EHRs for diabetic patients. Furthermore, the care teams are expected to consider behavioral health or psychosocial issues as potentially causal for any patient who suddenly worsens or stops adhering to their care plan. For patients who score positively on these mental health screening tests, CareMore physicians do not just refer them to a psychiatrist: as one senior physician administrator put it, "If we give patients a referral to a community-based psychiatrist for treatment of depression, they might get an appointment in 2 or 3 months if they are lucky. They need attention sooner than that."

Instead, CareMore created a behavioral health SWAT team composed of a psychiatrist, psychologist, and social worker who see a patient within 2 or 3 days of the positive screen in order to begin medications, cognitive behavioral therapy, or whatever else is needed. For the elderly patients who have become addicted to medications, the SWAT team often include an addiction specialist: "It was surprising to us. We have a lot of seniors who are addicted to prescription medications—sleeping pills, opioids—as well as to alcohol." At CareMore, as the management of chronic illness has become more standardized and efficient, intervening on the psychosocial and mental health issues has taken on ever-greater importance.

A fourth model of transformed behavioral healthcare comes from the for-profit company Quartet. Quartet believes that the approach followed by Advocate and Dr. Nagoshi's Central Medical Clinic—physically co-locating behavioral health specialists in each primary and specialty care office—is hard to scale and does not address the critical barriers to accessing behavioral healthcare.

Quartet's chief science officer, Dr. David Wennberg, argues that this model, called the collaborative care model, is useful but ultimately not a "perfect" solution:

> The data highlight a clear improvement in patient functional outcomes and reduced costs from Seattle's collaborative care model. But even after decades, this model hasn't spread everywhere. Why? It cannot scale. For structural, cultural, and logistical reasons, the expectation that we can "mass" co-locate behavioral health providers in primary care misses the mark. Furthermore, the collaborative care model is based on face-to-face visits. Some patients need alternatives. We need something else that works for patients and primary care physicians in their offices.

Quartet's alternative approach is called *virtual collaborative care*. The model uses technology to emulate the benefits of co-location, encouraging care coordination between primary care physicians, behavioral health specialists, and patients. The technology provides the healthcare team critical information regarding the patient, including behavioral assessment scores, appointment details, and post-appointment consultation notes to facilitate collaboration. The approach identifies patients with chronic medical illnesses who may have concurrent behavioral health conditions. It does this in 3 ways.

First, Quartet uses predictive modeling that reviews claims and other medical data to identify patients with diagnosed, undiagnosed, and latent behavioral healthcare issues. For example, Quartet may identify patients like Ms. Crawford with multiple emergency room visits whose primary diagnosis was chest or abdominal pain, but no confirmed physical ailment, as these patients might suffer from an underlying anxiety disorder or substance abuse.

Second, Quartet identifies patients who have had a behavioral health diagnosis but might not be optimally managed. Approximately 70% of patients with depression and other behavioral diagnoses do not receive effective treatments. Many have been started on medications but have never been assessed for adherence, optimal dosing, or their ongoing functional status and resolution of symptoms. Quartet stratifies patients, identifying those most in need of behavioral health interventions. The list of suggested patients is sent to the primary care physicians, who can then review Quartet's suggestions and decide whether to refer a patient for behavioral healthcare services.

Third, Quartet screens referred patients to further identify patients with potential undiagnosed behavioral health needs. If a patient presents with a behavioral health condition, they are then given a more detailed online assessment. Results are provided to the primary care physician and patient for review and discussion. This initial assessment serves as a baseline measure for future reference. Quartet then tries to reassess patients every 4 weeks to help evaluate the efficacy of both the interventions and the therapist interactions.

Once it is confirmed that a patient has a behavioral health issue, Quartet offers multiple solutions to best cater to their needs. The most common intervention is to refer a patient to a behavioral health specialist either via in-person therapy, virtual therapy, or computerized cognitive behavioral therapy. In instances and locations where a behavioral health specialist may not be readily available or desired, another option is a curbside consultation, which allows a primary care physician to speak with a psychiatrist within 15 minutes. This is typically done to help guide the physician in the adjustment of medication dosages or deciding the next steps in treatment. The physician is able to quickly address the patient's needs while also learning how to better manage behavioral health conditions.

For behavioral health referrals, Quartet attempts to ensure that patients receive the most appropriate care for the individual patient. To do so, Quartet's algorithm compiles a ranked list of potential behavioral health specialists each patient could see, taking into consideration diagnosis, preferred therapy modality (e.g., in person vs. virtual), insurance network, available times, zip code, quality and efficiency measures. After meeting with a patient, behavioral health specialists share a treatment plan with the patient's primary care physician. Approximately 40% to 50% of patients are seen by a behavioral health specialist within 10 to 14 days; those with more urgent needs are seen within 1 to 3 days.

About 70% of therapists involved with Quartet are licensed clinical social workers who work with psychiatrists to review referred patient treatment plans and escalate those in need to psychiatric care. Quartet does not specify how therapy should be used after a patient is matched, but therapists are urged to implement goal-focused therapy aimed at patient improvement in less than 6 months. To further incentivize high-quality care and address behavioral health access issues, select therapists are offered performance bonuses based on demonstrated improvement in patient-reported outcomes. Quartet offers providers a value-based payment model to drive evidence-based practices and support the nonreimbursed activities that often accompany collaborative care.

The Quartet team regularly assesses patients and provides feedback data to expedite outcomes improvements. Data measurement is a persistent challenge in behavioral health, a field in which disease improvement is still rarely assessed and treatment is often not appropriately escalated.

Quartet also provides primary care physicians with a reliable, efficient solution for their patients with behavioral health conditions. Gone are the days when primary care physicians' staff would spend hours attempting to find a psychiatrist or alternative behavioral healthcare for patients. Physicians do not need to create partnerships or formal affiliations with behavioral health specialists to ensure good care for their patients; instead, by partnering with Quartet, physicians can obtain high-value behavioral healthcare without the physician having to pay for or provide office space.

Behavioral health specialists receive higher volumes of appropriate patient referrals through Quartet, participate in value-based payments, and form closer working relationships with primary care physicians. Because Quartet uses virtual warm hand-offs, patient screenings, and standardized pre-visit assessments, its referral process results in fewer no-shows and higher revenue opportunities for behavioral specialists. Similar to primary care physicians, Quartet also provides behavioral health specialists with data on their patients' reported functional outcomes—something that has, until recently, been absent in the behavioral healthcare field.

Quartet provides patients with a curated group of convenient behavioral health specialists who are linked to their primary care physicians and who they can see with relatively short wait times. Quartet tracks outcomes so that adjustments to patients' therapeutic treatments can be made if there is insufficient improvement. A concierge service also supports patients to help troubleshoot common scheduling and accessibility challenges. Finally, Quartet offers a kind of shared decision making to help patients choose their type of therapeutic modality—whether face-to-face, virtual therapy, or some combination of the 2.

Quartet is currently operating in 4 cities, with approximately 1,500 behavioral health specialists included in its network. They have contracts with Steward Health Care System in Boston, Highmark Blue Cross Blue Shield in Pittsburgh, Premera Blue Cross in Seattle, and Humana in New Orleans. In the near future Quartet plans to expand into California with a leading health system and into New Jersey with an insurer.

Despite its initial success, Quartet has faced challenges. Its primary issue has been integrating its technology within primary care physicians' EHRs. Quartet hopes to eventually incorporate its assessments and treatment plans directly into the physician EHR in order to reduce barriers to rapid referrals and feedback on patients' therapeutic progress.

As with almost every recent behavioral health initiative, Quartet is still in the experimental phase. Its model is being refined. Quartet is currently studying whether its model of virtual collaborative care is as

good as face-to-face care and co-location of behavioral health specialists in physician offices based on patient outcomes. Although the company is still too young to demonstrate total cost of care reductions, the
early data is encouraging. The rate of missed first appointments with a
behavioral health specialist is much lower through Quartet, at just 15%,
compared to the national average of 40%. In addition, emergency room
visits appear to be declining for Quartet-supported patients. Anecdotal
evidence from Quartet in Massachusetts also suggests small declines in
total cost of care.

As physician practices and health systems master chronic care coordination, one area that will receive ever-greater attention is behavioral health. As a recent survey published in the journal *Health Affairs*
showed, there is "substantial interest in integrating behavioral healthcare into primary care across a majority of ACOs." This is in part because the mandate to screen for depression, anxiety, and other behavioral health problems has become the norm. However, such screening
needs to be accompanied by "an effector arm," a solution to ensure effective treatment for patients who screen positive. The fact that physicians are increasingly being held responsible for total cost of care also
bolsters interest in behavioral health. Therefore, providers now have an
interest in treating behavioral health problems early on in the hopes
of measurably lowering costs of chronically ill patients with comorbid
depression, anxiety, and substance abuse disorders.

Today many experiments are trying to identify the right way to deliver behavioral healthcare. Some approaches focus on co-locating
behavioral health specialists in primary care physicians' offices. Other
approaches connect primary care providers with behavioral health
providers who have unused appointments, allowing patients to be seen
promptly and behavioral health providers to increase their incomes.
Regardless of the type of intervention, these are early days. All these
models are still in the experimental stage of development. Over time
the truly effective practices will be identified. I believe that by 2020,
once chronic care coordinators have become routine, behavioral health
interventions will become a healthcare priority and will be standardized across the nation. By 2025, healthcare will be an effective balance
between behavioral healthcare and medical care—to the great benefit
of all Americans.

PRACTICE 10: HOME AND PALLIATIVE CARE

In her 73 years, Mrs. Eula Winston has seen the birth of 10 grandchildren and 4 great-grandchildren. She has held multiple jobs over the past 40 years. Mrs. Winston owned a daycare, worked as a domestic cleaning homes, and even had a stint as a home caregiver to homebound people. Most recently, Mrs. Winston volunteered at the primary school across the street from her home.

One year ago, Mrs. Winston experienced loss of appetite followed by diarrhea upon eating. After a few days she began feeling light-headed and became very dehydrated, so she went to the emergency room. The physicians discovered a blood clot in her lungs and multiple spots on her chest X-ray. They sat Mrs. Winston down and told her they suspected lung cancer.

Mrs. Winston was shocked by the diagnosis. Although she had once been a smoker, she had quit 35 years ago and had never experienced any shortness of breath or similar symptoms. She was transferred from her local hospital to one of Philadelphia's academic centers. A complete evaluation showed that she had metastatic lung cancer with lesions in the front right of her brain and in her spine. Mrs. Winston underwent a craniotomy to resect her brain lesion, followed by radiation therapy to both her brain and spine. While in the hospital Mrs. Winston experienced continued diarrhea and dehydration, but when they eventually resolved, she was discharged home.

About 3 months after her radiation, Mrs. Winston's back pain unexpectedly began to worsen. Tests at the hospital revealed that her spine lesions were growing. Once again, Mrs. Winston was admitted for pain control and even more radiation. She was then given chemotherapy with Tarceva (erotinib), an oral chemotherapy drug that interferes with specific growth-factor receptors on metastatic lung cancer cells. Ms. Winston was also prescribed a supportive care drug that works to reduce pain, fractures, and other problems from cancer that has spread to the bones. Today, Mrs. Winston is in the midst of her chemotherapy regimen, and what she hates the most is the rash and itching caused by the Tarceva, a common side effect. "It doesn't go away," she says. "It's not a good feeling. And the antibiotics they gave me made me sick with nausea and vomiting and sweats, so I stopped them." She does have some pain from the cancer, especially late at night and sometimes in the morning after she wakes up. "I have to take pain pills about 3 or 4 times a week. I take 'em before pain gets worse. It is never zero. But it's tolerable." Mrs. Winston does, however, like one of Tarceva's side effects, it makes her eyelashes grow very long. She gets lots of compliments about them, especially when she goes to church.

Upon meeting Mrs. Winston it is difficult to remember that this is a woman about to celebrate the one-year anniversary of her lung cancer diagnosis. That she made it this far is totally unexpected. After all, the median survival after brain metastases from lung cancer is only 4 months. Yet Mrs. Winston has not only beat the odds; she is living as though she were cancer-free. Her appetite is pretty good. She is out of the house 3 or 4 times per day, primarily to the supermarket and other shops. She is a Jehovah's Witness and goes to her Kingdom Hall twice a week: "I love it when I get there," she says. One week earlier, Mrs. Winston danced at a relative's wedding. She goes to plenty of appointments with her primary care physician, her cancer doctor, and radiation oncologist. Despite how active she is, Mrs. Winston does need help, especially with balance and taking a shower. Her daughter and, when they are in town, granddaughters, help sit her in the shower and wash up. Her granddaughter sums up Mrs. Winston's situation by saying that although she has some memory problems and can mentally go in and out, "she can't sit still."

Because patients with metastatic brain cancer have a short life expectancy, Mrs. Winston was referred to Aspire, a for-profit company that specializes in providing palliative but not hospice care to patients who have a life expectancy of one year or less. Aspire is the same company that sent McKenzie to Miss Harris after her fainting episode and the placement of her automatic implantable cardioverter defibrillator (see Chapter 1). Aspire works in 42 cities in 19 different states. Its model is to hire palliative care specialist physicians in each city who oversee and work with palliative care nurse practitioners. For patients, Aspire's model ensures they can stay at home and have access to care 24/7.

The nurse practitioners play a key role in Aspire's care delivery. Each one regularly visits their assigned patients in their homes. They address patients' symptoms and concerns up to the very last few weeks or even days of life. Initially, a primary focus of the nurse practitioner's visits is to help patients fill out an Advance Care Directive and a POLST form (Physicians Orders for Life-Sustaining Treatment). When Mrs. Winston's Aspire nurse practitioner first visited, she noticed that Mrs. Winston's Advance Care Directive was 6 years old. The nurse practitioner initiated a discussion to update the document. As Mrs. Winston tells the story, absentmindedly patting her documents, which rest on a folding table beside her, she becomes a little pensive:

> I'm afraid of dying. I know it is coming, but I try to get past that. I'm not going to think about it too much. I know it's going to happen sometime. But I'm doing good now.

As a Jehovah's Witness, Mrs. Winston refuses all blood transfusions. She doesn't want to be in the ICU and doesn't want any life-prolonging treatments such as respirators or dialysis.

As with Miss Harris, Mrs. Winston's Aspire nurse practitioner also ensures that she has—and properly takes—all the medications she needs. The day I am visiting Mrs. Winston, her nurse calls in to be sure a refill of Mrs. Winston's pain medications is sent to the house. She also checks in to be sure Mrs. Winston is eating and drinking enough and is getting the supportive care she needs. To ensure the family does not panic, call an ambulance, and launch a whole cascade of medical interventions, Aspire's nurse practitioner regularly reminds Mrs. Winston and her relatives of the process they have practiced, should something go wrong. "Call me on this number. Either I, or someone who works with me, will answer and make sure you get the right care." When patients like Mrs. Winston or Miss Harris inevitably progress—their symptoms get worse, they become totally bedbound, and get closer to death—Aspire will consult with the primary care physician to initiate hospice care.

What is amazing is that in the year since her diagnosis Mrs. Winston has been to the emergency room only once, when she was admitted to the hospital for 2 days because her tumor grew and caused serious problems. That is lower than the average 1-5 times a Medicare lung cancer patient is hospitalized, usually for 10 days total, in the last 6 months of life. Although Aspire's performance on cost and quality outcomes has not yet been subject to a formal, peer-reviewed study, it appears to be quite successful. For instance, 68% of Aspire's patients who die are enrolled in hospice for more than 3 days; its patients' median length of hospice is 41 days compared to national average of 17 days. Aspire patients have about half the hospital admissions in the last year of life compared to matched patients or patients in the system before Aspire started offering services. Both Miss Harris and Mrs. Winston are good examples of Aspire's success. By their own estimates, Aspire claims to save somewhere between 15% to 20% of costs for patients in the last year of life. Although these results remain to be confirmed by rigorous economic and quality-of-life analyses, they are nevertheless indicative of a potential breakthrough in improving end-of-life care with cost savings, succeeding in a field that has been marked only by disappointment for decades.

The Aspire model basically implements all the things end-of-life care experts have been advocating for several decades. It aims to begin palliative care interventions not in the last days or weeks of life, as so much of hospice does, but 12 months or more before death. This does not always work due in part to the vagaries of predicting life expectancy, but even its proposed intent is powerful. This allows patients and families to become comfortable with foregoing life-sustaining care, having effective symptom relief, and practicing calling the nurses rather than ambulances. It creates a sustained personal bond between one nurse practitioner and one patient ensuring that there is a trusting relationship when pivotal decisions need to be made. The Aspire model also focuses on discussing and documenting end-of-life care wishes, something physicians tend to find uncomfortable and thus avoid. The Aspire nurses are trained to initiate that dreaded conversation and direct it toward a practical end—completing the POLST form and an Advance Care Directive. It also aims to keep patients in their own homes, where patients want to be, toward the end of their lives. Finally, it is attractive because any physician practice or group can call Aspire. Practices do not have to build their own palliative care services, and can instead outsource the care to a trusted partner.

Effective, high-quality home care is becoming increasingly important. With greater de-institutionalization and with more attention to chronic care management, more patients will be receiving home care. Unfortunately, much of home care is poorly organized and delivered. Or as Clive Fields of VillageMD put it:

Most home care is uncoordinated and discombobulated. We have complicated patients with diabetes, congestive heart failure, emphysema, and renal disease needing a lot of care. They are often cared for by the specialists, who do not do a great job of coordinating the care. So they have someone coming to their house for blood draws. A separate person administering respiratory treatments. Someone else for wound care or changing their urinary catheter. And it drives the family crazy because someone has to basically quit their job and be home with the patient every day to coordinate with the home-care people.

Dr. Fields decided to change all that and created a separate division called Village@Home. The premise was simple but revolutionary: "We wanted to change from having multiple, single modality providers to having a single, multimodality provider." Instead of separate home-care providers for blood draws, wound care, physical therapy, respiratory therapy, and the rest, Village@Home empowered a nurse practitioner with extensive bedside experience to be the sole home-care provider. One person now can provide almost all the necessary patient services—writing prescriptions, drawing bloods, changing catheters, caring for wounds, administering breathing treatments, and the rest. The nurse practitioner teams up with a social worker for the patients who need social services.

Village@Home patients are typically those with complex chronic conditions or who are home bound, at high risk of readmission, or just have many needs. Others are identified by data analytics. And still others are recently discharged patients from hospitals and post-acute facilities. The Village@Home nurse practitioner has relatively longer visits with their patients. They see only 5 to 6 patients per day.

Recently Village@Home began expanding to help their affiliated specialists extend their services into the home, drawing specialty labs, providing wound care treatments, and even working with specialists to infuse medications, including cancer chemotherapy, at home. Clive Fields gives one example:

These oncologists were having patients with metastatic disease come to the office every week or every other week by ambulance to get a chemotherapy infusion. It was totally unnecessary and expensive care. And it was no good for the patient. Who wants to spend time going to an infusion suite when you could get the same treatment at home?

The Village@Home nurse can administer the chemotherapy right in the patient's home. It is not different than having a nurse do it at the infusion center. Our nurse practitioner can coordinate with the oncologist's office. And if this therapy is going to continue weekly until the patient dies, then it is much better for everyone.

Mark Lerner, who oversees Village@Home, gives another example:

Patients get transported by ambulance to the hospital for wound care. They get examined, bloods checked, wound debridement and magic dust sprinkled on their wounds, prescriptions refilled, and then taken by ambulance back home. The care is inconvenient and expensive and often the patient and family have no real idea what the goals of treatment are. And these typically are patients who are DNR [do not resuscitate], so much of this care is unnecessary.

One egregious example was a homebound, blind patient whose family was administering eye drops for glaucoma. The administration was painful and, since she was blind, totally unnecessary. We can send one nurse practitioner to the home and take care of it all—the wound care, any labs needed, and prescription renewals. She stopped the eye drops at once. Good home care just saves so much money and patient discomfort.

Clive Fields thinks this kind of relationship with specialists is likely to expand as payment changes:

Specialists have no capacity, and therefore no interest, in care outside of their office. They may provide great care in their office but are oblivious to what happens to a patient once they leave their office. But as more reimbursements move into capitated and other risk-bearing contracts, even specialists are looking to reduce overutilization, such as unnecessary ambulance rides, and improve the quality and cost of medical services. Village@Home can have one nurse doing all the appropriate care, instead of having them build their own infrastructure.

Village@Home transitions patients to Aspire when they need more specialized palliative care services.

Currently, under fee-for-service payment, Village@Home is breaking even. They are paid $85 per nurse practitioner home visit for 5 or 6 visits a day. But with capitation and financial risk, reducing ambulance rides, eliminating multiple home-care providers, and reducing unnecessary hospitalizations and readmissions, the Village@Home model could become a win-win-win—saving the system money, making money for home healthcare, and keeping patients in their own homes.

PRACTICE 11: COMMUNITY INTERVENTIONS

Lucas Downs is lying in a hospital bed, just itching to get out: "I just want to be away from here. I want to take my kids to Hawaii on vacation. Or to the mall to go shopping."

The past year had been a nightmare for Mr. Downs. One summer night just a year earlier, he was on his street in West Philadelphia when several men approached. He did not recognize them. The men, however, saw his bucket hat and mistook him for a foe. Fourteen bullets later, Mr. Downs was lying in a hospital, paralyzed from the waist down:

> I know I am blessed to see another day. Not too many people have been in my situation and are still here. My friend was shot with one bullet and died. I am trying to figure it out. God wanted to slow me down. Maybe I am here, alive, because I didn't deserve to be shot. Those guys mistook me for someone else. I am blessed to be here talking to you.

Mr. Downs may feel blessed to be alive, but he has hardly received optimal healthcare. After being stitched back together, he sat in bed for 24 hours every day. He developed bedsores on his buttock that refused to heal because he was not turned enough during his initial hospitalization and the subsequent 3 months of rehabilitation. He only received one week of physical therapy. Mr. Downs was also never given a cushion for his wheelchair. Once he returned home, Mr. Downs never received home care to help change the dressings covering his bedsores. He and his children never received any mental health or grief counseling after such a traumatic event. He never received any pain medication for the shooting pain caused by the sores; instead, the primary care physician initially assigned to Mr. Downs saw him once and then scheduled a follow-up . . . for one year later.

After being discharged from the rehabilitation facility, Mr. Downs returned to living with his mother in a walk-up. There was no ramp installed in the house. The only way he could get out of the house was to grab onto the banister and crawl with help from his mother and, sometimes, younger kids in the neighborhood. Getting out of the house proved incredibly difficult to do on a regular basis. Mr. Downs felt trapped.

During Mr. Downs's time at home the bedsores worsened and he began feeling lightheaded, dizzy, and weak. As he describes it, "I just didn't feel like myself." He eventually went to the emergency room. However, Mr. Downs became scared and angry when the physicians began discussing the need for surgery to mitigate the spread of the infection into his bones, and he thought he was not being taken care of quickly enough. He stormed out "Against Medical Advice." Upon coming home, however, his mother begged him to go back to the hospital. Mr. Downs eventually heeded her advice and returned.

This time the physicians quickly admitted Mr. Downs for sepsis—a bacterial infection in the blood stream—from his bedsores. During the hospitalization for sepsis something unusual happened. Ms. Cheryl, as Mr. Downs calls her, knocked on his hospital door to introduce herself. "She told me she was a community health worker," Mr. Downs explained, "and that she would be back to help me get everything I needed done." Ms. Cheryl lived up to her promise. She first helped organize a meeting between Mr. Downs, his family, and the medical team in order to facilitate communication and explain the need for surgery. After his healthcare team stabilized Mr. Downs, he was scheduled for a debridement surgery to clean the wounds and put in a skin flap over the exposed areas. The consent process and procedure went smoothly, as Ms. Cheryl made sure the team helped Mr. Downs understand what was happening along the way—and why.

Cheryl Garfield is a community health worker at the University of Pennsylvania Health System. What is a community health worker? They are not care coordinators for chronic care management who try to get patients to comply with their medical regimens—taking medications, checking their weight or glucose levels, exercising, getting their vaccines. Nor are they home health workers going to patients' homes to change bandages and administer breathing treatments and antibiotics. Instead, community health workers, who generally come from the same communities as their patients, help patients address the underlying social, financial, and behavioral causes of their health problems. They focus on the nexus between medical care and social services mainly for poorer patients with complex medical conditions and few social supports who would otherwise fall through the cracks.

At the University of Pennsylvania, the community health workers use the IMPaCT model, which recommends initiating an interaction by asking patients what *they* think will help them to become healthier. Working with patients, they create action plans covering 5 domains (see Table 6.1, page 231). Some of these involve health services, but most are centered on re-engaging the patients with their families and communities. Community health workers then help patients execute these plans.

Beyond the types of support community health workers provide, one other way of understanding this role is as providers of resources that enable patients to feel a sense of autonomy and control over their lives. By interacting with and focusing their attention on patients, community health workers communicate to the patients that someone cares about them and that they, too, are valuable people.

Mr. Downs is not the only patient Cheryl Garfield has worked with. Another memorable patient was Mr. Brenner, a 50-year-old man with a long history of abuse as a child. Mr. Brenner had served 9 months in jail for a charge of sexual assault but ultimately was never convicted. Although he had had a number of jobs, including as a manager at Walmart, Mr. Brenner's record made it hard for him to obtain higher-level positions. He had become socially isolated. Mr. Brenner fell into depression, tried to commit suicide multiple times, and was hospitalized 9 times in psychiatric facilities between 2012 and 2015. When Cheryl met Mr. Brenner, she used the semistructured interview style developed by the University of Pennsylvania Center for Community Health Workers to get to know her new patient. When she asked Mr. Brenner what gave him "joy in his life, or when had he last had fun or laughed," he said that nothing made him happy, and that "I only look forward to death." Yet after some more probing by Cheryl, he recalled enjoying going bowling many years before. So Cheryl, along with another colleague, took Mr. Brenner bowling. He had a wonderful time. He even laughed for the first time in years. Subsequently Cheryl helped him get health insurance, find a primary care physician at a city health center, meet with a nutritionist at the YMCA, and find subsidized housing. Today Mr. Brenner is no longer suicidal. In the 15 months since meeting Cheryl he has been to the hospital only once.

Community healthcare workers are used at Penn in 3 main ways. First, the transitions program enrolls patients who are being discharged from the hospital. The community health workers follow these patients for 2 to 4 weeks, ensuring they have the health and social services they need at home, that they go to their medical appointments, and that they become socially engaged. A main goal is to ensure appropriate medical follow-up in order to reduce readmissions. A second program has community health workers work with patients who came into the emergency room 3 or more times in the previous 6 months. These patients typically have trauma, mental health, or end-of-life care issues with insufficient social support systems. In this program the community health workers follow patients for up to 12 weeks. Finally, in the outpatient program community health workers identify patients in physician offices, enrolling those in low-income zip codes, on public insurance, and with 2 or more chronic conditions, one of which is in poor control. For example, some of the patients are dual-eligible patients with diabetes and asthma and whose hemoglobin A1c is over 9%. These patients are followed for up to 6 months.

The value of community health workers for a physician's office or health system is in improving outcomes and decreasing utilization for a poorer population that relies on social and community services. The main outcomes can include improving HCAHPS scores—a patient satisfaction survey tied to reimbursement bonuses—and improving patients' quality of life measures and objective health outcomes, such as control of hemoglobin A1c for diabetic patients. For health systems the main benefit may be financial, such as increased payment from improved HCAHPS scores and savings from both reduced 30-day readmissions and shifting the care of chronic conditions from the emergency room and hospital to outpatient clinics.

Many clinics and health systems have successfully created community health worker programs. But many have also failed. What makes the University of Pennsylvania's Center successful? According to Shreya Kangovi, the program's creator and medical director, and Jill Feldstein, the administrative director, there are 6 keys to success (see Table 6.2, page 232), but far and away the most important one is hiring. They are looking for a "people person." They tend not to focus on résumés and academic credentials and instead look for compassionate people who have shown dedication to community engagement and organizing. They want individuals who can listen and connect with people and have shown a desire to help. This was obvious when I was walking with Cheryl to Lucas Downs's hospital room. She walks briskly but immediately calls out, "Hi, Francis! How's it going?" to the person manning the front desk. Then, "You're looking good today" to the cleaning staff polishing the floors. As we move through the hospital Cheryl affirmatively acknowledges every single person she passes. Cheryl's coworkers are equally warm and passionate. They include Lisa, who worked in customer service for years and has a history of building relationships with the Elks, VFW, and a variety of other community organizations. Another worker, Tony, was the liaison between Philadelphia schools and the local community and drove the creation of youth cultural programs. In general, these community health workers are naturals at listening, making people feel at ease talking about themselves, and forging connections. They also get satisfaction out of solving people's problems—making things happen.

Additionally, the Penn Center for Community Health Workers does not just hire and then deploy its workers. It has developed a 104-hour, 4-week classroom training program intended to be interactive for adults, primarily by ensuring plenty of role playing. The training course is college accredited, so workers can receive credit toward a degree, should they wish to do so. The classroom work is then followed by 2 weeks of shadowing a senior health worker and 2 weeks of being shadowed by a senior worker as the new community health worker starts the process of independent patient engagement.

Although this training is important, Kangovi believes there are additional elements crucial to the model's success, such as the use of standardized protocols. These protocols, which include the semistructured interview techniques, help community health workers ask the right questions to get to know their patients. When Cheryl asked Mr. Brenner about joy and fun in his life, it was not ad hoc or a question that just happened to occur to her; rather, it is a standard question community health workers ask all patients.

Staff safety is another substantial priority for the program. Dr. Kangovi and Ms. Feldstein are not naïve do-gooders; they know they are working in some of the roughest zip codes in Philadelphia, often with patients who have criminal records, are subject to domestic violence, or have mental health issues. They want to not only ensure their staff can help their patients, but also that they always go home to their own families at the end of the day. For example, one community health worker learned that one of her patients was living under a death threat from a neighborhood gang. This triggered a "safety huddle" with her manager and program directors. The goal of the safety huddle is to collectively identify any threats to community health workers and create a clear plan for minimizing risk. In this case, they decided that the community health worker would not meet the patient in-person at his house or at any place other than the hospital or his primary care physician's office. Very rarely, however, the program has to say no; safety concerns may prohibit community health workers from being able to help. Nevertheless, the program works hard to try to find a solution whenever possible. Community health workers can meet patients one-on-one in public places, such as a restaurant, the YMCA, or a library. Home visits are also encouraged, but the community health worker must go with a buddy. As an additional safeguard, the project manager must check in every hour or so by calling each community health worker on a home visit with a patient.

Another important element of the model's success is the center's creation of an electronic workflow system that allows community health workers to document the goals of each patient interaction and to specify what they plan on doing for each client. This allows them to measure their outcomes and accomplishments.

Finally, the program has extensive supervision. A project manager—typically a social worker—supervises each community health worker. The manager and community health workers meet weekly to review the plan for each patient, establish realistic timelines, assess progress toward the goals, and brainstorm about how to overcome obstacles. Additionally, the meeting allows the community health worker to debrief, cope with stress related with patient visits, and find their own support network.

The Penn Center has treated over 5,000 patients like Lucas Downs and Mr. Brenner since 2012. It has rigorously evaluated its program, documenting significantly improved HCAHPS scores, improvement in mental health outcomes, an approximate 3.5% absolute reduction in hospital admissions and readmissions, and a financial return of $2 to $1 invested in the program.

More importantly, the patients are fans of the program. Lucas Downs likes Cheryl. "I like to call her just to talk," Mr. Downs says. "I will definitely keep in touch with Ms. Cheryl after she stops being my community health worker." And Cheryl has been good for more than just talk. She helped Mr. Downs get a cushion for his wheelchair and a ramp for his home. Cheryl connected Mr. Downs to a new primary care doctor whom Mr. Downs trusts. As a result, he is now more compliant with his medical treatments—allowing nurses to do their work, including changing his bandages and "sticking me with needles." He is also getting mental health counseling. But Mr. Downs is especially looking forward to Cheryl helping him go to the mall and, given that he was always athletic, finding a place to play wheelchair basketball.

The Community Health Workers program could be expanded beyond the 3 main areas currently used by the University of Pennsylvania. For instance, like the Nurse-Family Partnership programs, it could also focus on prenatal care for pregnant women and the first year after delivery. Additionally, the program could expand beyond just poor patients with multiple medical problems to include any patient who is socially isolated and might need help navigating the challenges of life with chronic illness.

The key to transforming healthcare lies in part in establishing a systematic program like the one at the University of Pennsylvania, one that clearly delineates the functions of the workers and has a structured way of deploying and supervising them. The program needs this structure and focus in order to produce both financial and health returns for the medical side of the equation—the practice and health system—as well as health and psychosocial improvements for the patient side.

PRACTICE 12: LIFESTYLE INTERVENTIONS

I began the Nifty after Fifty exercise program because I was looking at data on our patients and noticed a lot of hip fractures, head lacerations, and other problems related to falls. I thought we could reduce these problems through strength training. Starting at age 40, we lose almost 1% of our muscle strength each year, and that increases to about 1.5% in our 60s. Most of us are half as strong at 80 as we were when we were 40. Similarly our ability to remember things peaks at age 25 and then declines.

I thought lifestyle changes and customized fitness training could help slow or stop these declines. So I started by taking 12 members to the YMCA twice a week and doing exercises with them. After the YMCA started asking for more money to use their facilities, we moved to L.A. Fitness. Eventually we built a facility adjacent to one of our care centers so patients could go directly from the physician's office to exercise.

So explains Sheldon Zinberg, the creator of CareMore's Nifty after Fifty exercise facilities and programs. In 1993, Zinberg created Care-More, and he remained the founding chairman until 2006, when he sold it and focused exclusively on Nifty after Fifty. Today Nifty after Fifty is a separate, distinct company. It is not owned by Anthem, Care-More's current owner, but still works in partnership with CareMore as well as other health systems. Since its founding in 2003 the Nifty after Fifty program has expanded to 38 facilities, with over 1 million patient visits per year.

When you enter a Nifty after Fifty facility, you immediately notice how different it is from your average gym. There are no sleek mirrors or high-end machines; no toned, youthful gym fanatics wearing tight, body-hugging spandex; and no large-screen TVs broadcasting the most recent football game or CNN. "If people are watching TV while they are exercising," Zinberg explains, "they might be distracted and not pay attention to proper exercise form or they might trip and get hurt by the machine." The average Nifty after Fifty center is home to seniors in loose-fitting clothes, machines for strength training that facilitate seated workouts, and seated bikes and steppers for aerobics. In the background plays music from the 1950s and 1960s, when the members were teenagers.

Instead of treadmills and free weights, there is an array of pneumatic resistance exercise equipment, similar to what you might find in collegiate or professional sports teams' weight rooms, designed to reduce impact-related injuries. No one is waiting for a machine to open up nor does any machine sit idle—seniors schedule a specific time during which they will come to Nifty after Fifty, which is open 10 hours a day, starting around 6 in the morning. Kinesiologists trained in geriatrics hover around the equipment and work with the clients. Each facility has 1 kinesiologist for every 12 participants.

In an adjacent room, 12 seniors sit in chairs and play "No Fall Volleyball" under the supervision of a kinesiologist. The players must follow all the usual rules of the game, plus one more—they cannot get up from their seats. This limited mobility encourages twisting, which builds abdominal and core strength without risking falls and improves hand-eye coordination. The room hosts other group exercise classes, such as yoga and Zumba, and physical therapy services. As the volleyball game wraps up, one 81-year-old player proudly proclaims that he attends Nifty after Fifty classes 5 times a week. His only complaint? That the volleyball should feature more frequently on the schedule.

A key component of Nifty after Fifty is that a kinesiologist initially evaluates each senior in order to design a customized workout routine. Zinberg is a strong proponent of this customization, as it is vital to targeting each senior's specific weaknesses in order to reduce the risk of specific injuries. For instance, although one person with diabetic foot drop and another with weak hip flexors are both at risk of falls, they are at risk for very different reasons and therefore require distinct exercise routines to strengthen specific muscle groups. Each member's customized routine is loaded onto a personal key, which can be inserted into the machines. The machine will then display the repetitions that the kinesiologist prescribed for the senior as well as the target power for each exercise. The key also enables tracking of each member's fitness progression. Outside of the physical facilities, Nifty after Fifty members are given exercises to perform at home. Through the use of such customized workouts, Zinberg believes the health and well-being of seniors can be significantly improved.

Although Nifty after Fifty initially began as a fall-prevention program, it has evolved into much more. It offers an Encore Heart Health program that serves as a prediabetic prevention program as well as programs for patients with specific chronic diseases. Today Nifty after Fifty facilities offer both tailored workouts and group counseling on diet and cooking. The benefits from such resources, in addition to exercise, are compounded by the program's psychosocial function. Zinberg notes that friendships, relationships, and even marriages have all grown out of Nifty after Fifty. The program plays such a significant role in members' lives that one senior even asked to have his memorial service there:

> I had a guy bench pressing 100 pounds 10 times, 3 sets. He had been coming here for around 4 years. He died at 96, and he wrote a note to his wife that he wanted a memorial service at Nifty. And we did it on a Saturday afternoon.

When Nifty after Fifty first began, Zinberg evaluated the program by comparing the rates of falls, hospitalizations, hip replacements, and other medical complications over 18 months between those seniors participating in the exercise program and those on the waiting list. In order to ensure impartiality, Zinberg asked staff unrelated to the program to undertake the research. "We had secretaries who had no idea what they were looking at," Zinberg explains, "pull the total medical services of the different patients and compare them." The secretaries estimated that among the many savings that resulted from the program, the average nights of hospitalization per person participating in the program compared to those on the waiting list were reduced by 1 and the average use of skilled nursing facilities was reduced by 1.4 days—decreases that alone amounted to savings of nearly $3,000 per person. These savings were achieved at a monthly cost for the program of about is $40 (or $500 per year) per person. Zinberg argues that "while any exercise is better than no exercise at all, an individually customized and computer-monitored progressive program to improve overall fitness achieves the best results. This is true whether the person is a frail elderly or a healthy and energetic senior."

Nifty after Fifty caters to the frail elderly cohort characteristic of CareMore. Therefore, it is not for vibrant seniors who *do* want an environment full of flashing TVs and spandex workout clothes. Nifty after Fifty is successful, but only to a point. Perhaps in acknowledgement of its limited marketability, CareMore is hoping to add more exercise options that could cater to a wider demographic of seniors. And Nifty after Fifty is developing a "Fitness Everywhere" program that combines traditional gym membership with experienced kinesiologists who will perform thorough fitness evaluations and design customized workouts.

Nevertheless, the program is unique: other health systems offer nothing nearly as extensive as Nifty after Fifty. One program that comes close, however, lies 2,800 miles across the United States in Westchester, New York. WESTMED also focuses on fall prevention, though they have opted for free tai chi classes rather than in-house gyms:

> When patients get their fall-prevention screening, we divide them into groups . . . [those at risk of falls] are welcome at our free tai chi classes. We are running about 8 to 10 sessions a week in 2 of the large polyclinic facilities. They are sold out and there's a waiting list.
>
> Published results have shown that tai chi has a 5 to 1 return in terms of reducing fall risks. Since WESTMED's investment in its tai chi classes is minimal, this program is essentially a "freebie," creating large returns from little investment.

Shamokin, Pennsylvania, is coal country. First settled around the time of the Revolutionary War, its fate has been tied to coal ever since. Its population is 98.8% white. The median household income is about 70% of the national average, and unemployment is about 20% higher than the national average. In the local schools, 80% of the children are on free or reduced breakfast and lunch. Fewer students graduate from high school or go on to college than the national or even Pennsylvania average. In the 2016 presidential election, over 69% of the votes in Shamokin went for Trump.

Like many such places, Shamokin's health statistics are poor. James, a 56-year-old resident, is not atypical. He is 6-foot-3 and weighs 474 pounds. He has diabetes that is out of control; his hemoglobin A1c hovers around 9.5% (normal is under 7.0%). Several years ago, Andrea Feinberg, a critical care internist, moved from Los Angeles and a faculty position at UCLA to a town near Shamokin when her husband became CEO of Geisinger Health System. Before she figured out what she wanted to do, she volunteered in the local community, working with a food bank to fill backpacks with food to ensure food-insecure children are fed through the weekend. She said

> I was horrified by the food we were giving them. It was all processed food with high sugar and carbohydrate content. Empty calories just to stave off hunger. It was poisonous. If I won't give this stuff to my children, I felt I shouldn't give it to someone else's children. And if I kept doing this, soon enough we would be treating these kids for diabetes.

The problem was that the food banks had only $1 to $2 per child per weekend to spend on food. What to do?

It occurred to Dr. Feinberg that the residents of Shamokin were strapped for cash. Paradoxically, this might make them more receptive to changing their diets. "I figured if they were given healthy food, they would not buy a Snickers bar, but would eat the good food and take the money they saved and pay their electric bill or buy gas for their car or pay the rent." Maybe by giving people in Shamokin healthy food instead of the unhealthy processed food, it would be possible to change diets and the trajectory of diabetes in part because their low incomes limited their options.

She went to one Geisinger clinic that serves about 6,000 patients. Patients do not have to be members of Geisinger to still get care at the clinic. Dr. Feinberg analyzed the clinic's population and identified all the patients with out-of-control diabetes—that is, with hemoglobin A1c over 8.0%. She then determined which ones were food insecure, defined as whether they ran out of money to buy food at or before the end of the month, or were worried they might run out of food itself. Then she conducted a small pilot study and scaled it up to 60 patients—1% of the clinic's population. Each patient had to participate in a 6-week course—2.5 hours per week—that educated them on diabetes and self-management. They also met with a dietician who taught them recipes and menus. Each week they also received a "food prescription" that included 3 grocery bags of fresh fruits, fresh vegetables, whole grains, and lean protein such as chicken, fish, and the occasional pork or ground turkey. Every 2 weeks they also received eggs, whole wheat bread, oats, and milk for breakfasts. The food was enough for 10 meals—not just for the patient but for the entire household. The thinking was that if one patient was an out-of-control diabetic, others in the household were more likely to be diabetic, prediabetic, or at risk. The educational sessions occurred on the days they picked up the food. Patients were also encouraged to exercise, building up vigorous walking from 1 minute per day to 30 minutes per day. There was no cost to the patients.

There was 100% compliance—everyone came every week to pick up their food. After 12 weeks, James's hemoglobin A1c dropped from 9.6% to 7.7%, and he lost 30 pounds. Another woman's hemoglobin A1c dropped from 10.0% to 8.0%. Not only did she lose 35 pounds, but she also got a nicotine patch and began to quit smoking, dropping from 3 packs to 5 cigarettes per day, even though the program does not include anything about smoking. There was only one major problem: hypoglycemia—low blood sugars. Ironically, as the patients ate better and exercised, their glucoses were under better control but they kept taking the same amount of insulin. This made them overshoot.

Weis Markets, a fixture in central Pennsylvania, has largely funded the program because the 3rd-generation owner is committed to investing in the local community and healthy living. The cost for the food is roughly $25 per household per week, or $1,300 per year. This is not insignificant. Dr. Feinberg wants to find out whether it is possible to recoup those costs in improved health and reduced medical bills. As Geisinger expands the program, it will be rigorously evaluated to quantify the health outcomes as well as the economics by measuring the impact on the use of the emergency room, the number of hospitalizations, and the total cost of the patients' care. But given how few interventions have worked to change diet and obesity, Dr. Feinberg's experiment is very encouraging. Its insight that lower-income Americans, ones at risk for diabetes, might also be more receptive to altering their diets is the kind of innovative thinking that is needed in the area of lifestyle interventions.

There is probably nothing so difficult as trying change a patient's lifestyle. The frequency of broken New Year's resolutions attests to how hard it is for any of us to change our lifestyle habits. Finding time to fit in exercise or learning how to cook differently or foregoing sugar, salt, and processed foods is hard. Nevertheless, many transformed practices, groups, and health systems have begun introducing lifestyle interventions that are promising. They typically begin with free tai chi or other exercise programs, because the return on investment is clear—preventing falls and broken hips saves money by reducing the number of $25,000 hip replacements. And even at $500 per patient per year, $25,000 savings translates into needing just 1 forestalled operation for every 50 high-risk patients. As other effective interventions to alter lifestyle habits are created and tested, such as Geisinger's healthy food initiative, they will need to generate health improvements and cost savings to make them sustainable. The most transformed practices and groups see great value not just in providing higher-quality and lower-cost medical services, but also in changing lifestyles to forestall the need for medical services. Over the next decade, such innovative practices will move from experiments to routines at transformed medical organizations.

HEALTHCARE IN the United States has passed a tipping point. Now everyone accepts the need for transforming the delivery system to provide patient-centric, value-based, and population-based care, thereby fulfilling the triple aim.

By studying a wide variety of physician practices, multispecialty groups, and health systems from New York to Hawaii, I have distilled 12 transformational practices to show, in some detail, what it takes to make that kind of difference. By describing specific examples, I have identified what differentiates the successful from failed attempts for the better-known transformational practices such as chronic care coordination.

Chapter 8 discusses how medical organizations starting on the transformational journey should begin implementing these practices. Before that, however, I survey a practice that receives significant attention but is not essential to transforming the delivery of care. The next chapter explores why virtual medicine, despite plenty of hype and investment, is not currently—and unlikely to be in the foreseeable future—integral to the transformation and delivery of high-quality and low-cost care.

Chapter 7

VIRTUAL MEDICINE

A Red Herring?

THE PROMISE OF VIRTUAL MEDICINE

It was a hot but not humid early September day. Mr. Brenner braved the heat to drive to the Clinical Decision Unit of one of Kaiser Permanente Mid-Atlantic "Hubs." These units are a combination of urgent care, a procedure suite, and a 24-hour observation suite. They have all the typical diagnostic services of a hospital—laboratory, ultrasound, CT, and other imaging modalities—and even negative pressure rooms for patients suspected of having tuberculosis or other highly contagious infections. During extended business hours, they are typically staffed by board certified internists, family practitioners, and emergency medicine physicians.

Mr. Brenner arrived complaining of a rash and joint pain. Because the unit was busy, Mr. Brenner was offered the opportunity to do a "video visit" with a unit physician from a neighboring Kaiser Permanente Hub who had some free time. The video visit would be in a dedicated exam room with a Cisco system that had a camera, large-monitor video otoscope for looking in the throat or ears, and video stethoscope for listening to the lungs or heart. And there would be no wait and no copay for this visit. To Mr. Brenner, this sounded like a good deal. He opted for the virtual visit with the remote physician, named Dr. Kim.

During their high-fidelity video chat, Mr. Brenner explained when he noticed the rash and joint pain. Dr. Kim asked a number of questions. After a few minutes of talking Dr. Kim asked him to take the special camera with the light and point it toward the rash so Dr. Kim could take a closer look. After conducting this virtual physical exam, Dr. Kim rendered his diagnosis and told Mr. Brenner he was ordering a Lyme titer. And just like that, Mr. Brenner's ailments were attended to.

Listen to the medical techno-utopians or commentators like Eric Topol and you hear of a future in which Mr. Brenner's virtual visit is just the tip of the iceberg. All medicine, these analysts proclaim, will become virtual medicine. Healthcare will be dominated by wearable technologies that continuously monitor key physiological and other indicators, from blood pressure and glucose to heart rhythms and physical activity, and then send that information back to monitoring sites. Other electronic monitors will assess medication compliance, peak respiratory flows, weight, and even mood. Like Mr. Brenner's experience, almost every interaction between a patient and a physician or other clinician will be a virtual visit conducted from wherever the patient happens to be over the Web. There will be little need for the patient and healthcare team to ever physically meet or interact. Peter Kuhn, a professor of medicine at USC, has strongly urged for this virtual shift:

> The more than 30,000 minutes between visits are a missed opportunity. Technology can be leveraged to fill this gap and provide a comprehensive picture [of the patient]. The collected data [from wearable technologies] can lead to better treatment decisions, better survival rates, and better understanding between physician and patient.

The real techno-utopians go even further. They think that the notion of a human physician is also quaint. Watson or some better machine learning computer will be able to monitor the physiological and other data in real time, create a list of potential diagnoses, zero in on the most probable diagnosis, and provide the best treatments. And who knows, many techno-utopians think soon computers will even be able to perform necessary surgical procedures.

If that *is* the future, it is probably far, far—even decades—away. Indeed, it is unlikely to become our reality. Today, virtual medicine is in its infancy. More importantly, it is not a core of transformation practice—and it is unlikely to become one in the next decade. Currently, most innovative physician offices and health systems, such as Kaiser Permanente, are using some telemedicine and remote monitoring. These systems have found it to be helpful, as it is convenient for both physicians and patients. Virtual medicine probably could and will be expanded in the near future. But there are still plenty of kinks. And the current evidence is decidedly negative on the overall impact of virtual medicine on health outcomes. More importantly, virtual medicine—whether by video and remote electronic monitoring or by wearables—appears to be, at best, useful only in augmenting a few elements of an already transformed patient care experience. It itself it is not transformative in the ways techno-utopians imagine.

Virtual medicine is not what practices or health systems should invest in for the first or second stages of their transformations. Indeed, virtual medicine can only supplement, but never completely replace, face-to-face clinician-patient interactions. It is—and for the foreseeable future will be—most useful in providing physicians and other healthcare providers with actionable information. Virtual medicine should be invisible to patients rather than the heart of clinician-patient interactions. As Lee Sacks of Advocate stated, it is best "working in the background."

At Kaiser Permanente Mid-Atlantic, video visits like Mr. Brenner's can be done on a computer, tablet, or smartphone. They are available for regular office visits with a patient's primary care physician and for virtual house calls for urgent care—but never for emergency care. The typical virtual "house call" is from a working mother who can only call at 8 or 9 p.m., once dinner is done, the children are in bed, and the house is straightened up. The mother can then finally get around to her own self-care and usually calls in asking about flu-like symptoms, unusual menstrual bleeding, and other common concerns. These virtual visits are also useful for real-time consultations. For instance, pediatric subspecialists or dermatologists who are scarce can cover a wide area from the comfort of their own office.

Another, somewhat surprising use for video visits is for psychiatric care. At Kaiser Permanente a psychotherapist is available 24/7 via video. The virtual therapist is useful for patients with agoraphobia—an anxiety disorder characterized by fear of public places or public embarrassment—and for those feeling an impending crisis resulting from depression. The therapist can talk to the patients, provide care, and make an immediate triage decision.

CareMore is another a player in the field of virtual medicine. The system distributes wireless blood pressure cuffs to hypertensive patients, wireless scales to congestive heart failure patients, and wireless glucose monitors to diabetic patients. These can be helpful in monitoring patients who are newly diagnosed with their condition or who, for whatever reason, are not regularly self-reporting their results.

THE REAL—MINOR—IMPACT OF VIRTUAL MEDICINE

Kaiser Permanente and CareMore are at the most advanced stages of transformation. Yet even for them, virtual medicine is a relatively minor part of their care. Its role is so small, in fact, that it does not significantly contribute to their transformations in care. At best, virtual medicine might be considered exploratory or experimental. For instance, fewer than 1% of all patient touch-points at Kaiser are conducted via live or 2-way video visits. Dr. Bernadette Loftus, the associate director of Kaiser Permanente Medical Group, Mid-Atlantic region, noted that in the years they have used virtual medicine—since 2011—it may have saved 10 to 15 physician hires from among their 1400 physicians, resulting in a savings of about 1%.

Many start-ups, such as Doctor on Demand, are now entering the virtual medicine field with high hopes. After receiving the public recognition of Dr. Phil, Doctor on Demand saw 1 million visits last year alone. That sounds like a lot. As a business opportunity, 1 million visits may be profitable, but it is ultimately a tiny fraction of the nearly 1 billion physician office visits and 136 million emergency room visits that occur each year in the United States, not to mention the who knows how many telephone calls to healthcare providers.

The real question is not about how often virtual medicine is used, but whether it makes an actual difference in improving healthcare outcomes. At Kaiser Permanente, Dr. Loftus has asked just this question. She wants to know empirically whether virtual medicine improves outcomes, such as blood pressure and glucose control, and whether it is efficient, actually saving time for physicians and other providers and thereby reducing per-unit costs. At the moment younger, tech-savvy Kaiser members and those with children who find the technology "cool" seem to like using the video visits. Yet by lowering the barriers to accessing physicians and other clinicians, virtual medicine may cater to the "worried well," giving them one more way to bombard healthcare teams with their fears. Ironically, this could end up increasing physician workloads while not actually improving the overall health of Kaiser's patient population—a lose-lose situation. Dr. Loftus has decided that she wants firm data before embarking on a significant expansion of Kaiser Permanente's virtual medicine program.

The evidence that *does* exist is not tremendously encouraging. Studies trying to integrate wearables, electronic monitors, and other virtual medicine technologies into medical practice have generally failed to improve patient outcomes. Three recent studies give a flavor for the failures of virtual medicine. A research group from the University of Pittsburgh tried to use virtual technology to enhance weight-loss interventions for 471 young adult patients (aged 18 to 35) who ranged from overweight to obese (BMIs ranging from 25 to 40). All patients were on a low-calorie diet, were prescribed increased physical activity (100 minutes per week of moderate physical activity, which increased over time to 300 minutes per week), and were enrolled in weekly group counseling sessions. After 6 months, all patients participated in telephone counseling sessions, received text message prompts, and were given access to materials on a website that offered a new behavioral tip each week. Half of the patients were randomized to the technology-enhanced group and were given a multisensor wearable device. The device wrapped around the upper arm and provided feedback to the participant on physical activity and energy expenditure, both through a display and by linking to a website. The website also allowed self-monitoring of dietary intake. After 24 months, the control group lost an average of over 13 pounds—or 6.3% of their body weight. The technology-enhanced group lost under 8 pounds—3.6% of their body weight. Perhaps the basic intervention was so good that the patients' weight loss was prohibitively high, making technology enhancement incapable of really improving on the outcome. However, the researchers had to admit that "the addition of wearable technology to a behavioral intervention was less effective for 24-month weight loss." Virtual medicine performed worse on a real health outcome than no technology at all.

In another study, adult employees from 13 companies in Singapore were divided into 4 groups to test whether wearable technology would increase physical activity and impact weight loss, blood pressure, and other health outcomes. The control group received no intervention. Another group was given Fitbit Zip activity trackers. A third group was given the Fitbit with an additional incentive of a charitable donation should a patient increase his or her physical activity. The final group was given the Fitbit and a cash incentive. At 6 months those groups with the Fitbit and either a charity contribution or cash incentives did increase their moderate-to-vigorous physical activity by 20 to 30 minutes per week—a statistically significant amount and an important step toward the goal of the 150 minutes per week of moderate physical activity recommended by the CDC. After 6 months, the incentives were discontinued but people were allowed to keep the Fitbit. When measured at 6 and 12 months, patients using wearable technologies showed "no improvements in any health outcomes (weight, blood pressure, etc.) ... calling into question the value of these devices for health promotion." The researchers also noted that the wearable alone was not helpful; instead, it had to be combined with other incentives to provide meaningful change, substantially increasing the cost of such virtual medicine interventions.

A third study aimed to change the outcomes for nearly 1500 chronically ill patients aged 50 years and above (on average 73 years of age) who were hospitalized with congestive heart failure (CHF) exacerbations. These are precisely the types of high-cost, chronically ill patients whose patterns of care need to be changed the most if the system is going to produce consistently higher quality and lower costs—the primary focus of any transformed delivery system (see Chapter 4, pages 93–106). Upon hospital discharge patients either received usual care or a virtual medicine intervention consisting of wireless electronic cuffs that measured blood pressure and heart rate, wireless scales, and digital symptom monitoring. The patients were asked to use the cuffs, scales, and other machines daily. The physiological data were sent to a centralized call center where nurses monitored the patients and, following a defined protocol and called patients when readings exceeded a specific threshold. The nurses asked about potential causes of the abnormal readings, and "when symptoms were concerning, patients were encouraged to contact their health professionals." Overall, slightly over half of the patients used the virtual medicine machines 50% or more of the time. Interestingly, during the 6-month period each patient triggered a nurse alert an average of 22 times—a nontrivial workload burden. Over the same 6 months, about 50% of patients were hospitalized with another congestive heart failure exacerbation, and nearly 15% died. Ultimately, the electronic monitoring technologies and nurse interventions made no difference. As the University of California researchers concluded, the study "found that a combination of remote [electronic] patient monitoring with care transition management did not reduce 180-day all-cause readmission after hospitalization for [congestive heart failure]. [In addition,] 180-day mortality was also not reduced with the intervention."

Maybe the best overall assessment of virtual medicine comes from Dr. Andrew Schutzbank, vice president of Iora Health, an innovative primary care start-up operating 13 practices in 6 states. "I have no use for a continuous blood pressure monitor for a patient walking around," Dr. Schutzbank has stated. "I have once- or at best twice-a-day medications that work over hours. Knowing the minute-to-minute changes in blood pressure is totally unhelpful unless I am managing the patient in the ICU." As for virtual office visits using a smartphone or computer, he considers them glorified telephone calls. He believes that half of the time the technology does not even work, and the other half of the time it frustrates both the physician and patient. At Iora, the most useful virtual medicine technology is, by a wide margin, secure text messaging for follow-up care. Although these communications allow patients to convey how their symptoms are progressing and allow physicians to respond accordingly, they also offer a sense of personal connections. Dr. Schutzbank has found that many patients are often texting their physicians about their pets, their daily activities, or just to say hello.

VIRTUAL MEDICINE AND PATIENT CONVENIENCE

One of the strongest arguments for virtual medicine is patient convenience. Patients can contact their physician, nurse practitioner, care manager, or a clinician who has access to their electronic health records from the comfort of their own home. They can ask a quick question by email. They can talk through a video link so the physician can get a good gestalt about how sick they look. They can show a dermatologist the rash or skin mole that is worrying them. This allows people to get care without dressing up, traveling 30 minutes, waiting in the office or urgent care facility, paying for parking, and driving back home. Virtual medicine can short circuit all of that and make what used to be an onerous experience as convenient as online shopping.

But convenience can be a double-edged sword. Virtual medicine does allow patients to contact their physicians with minimal effort, which, as I have noted, can enhance access for patients. Patients with behavioral health problems such as agoraphobia can receive care from a specialist. Dermatologists can diagnose many more skin conditions. And many people do not have to brave the elements in the middle of the night to get attention for urgent problems, such as a child with a high fever, that are not life threatening and therefore do not necessitate a physical visit to the emergency room.

But convenience can also be a major problem. By reducing barriers to contacting physicians, the worried well can consume a lot of valuable physician and nurse time with minor or even nonexistent health problems. They can use access to physicians or nurse practitioners in lieu of searching the Web. At Kaiser Permanente I was told of how mothers use the virtual medicine portals because their technology-infatuated children like using the video link and talking to the physician through the computer. Similarly, at Dean Clinic physicians complain bitterly about the dramatic increase in the volume of emails and text messaging along with the patients' expectations that they would get a response before the end of the business day. One noted,

> With email, we've opened Pandora's box. The average pediatrician has something like 2,500 high-complexity email, phone message, and other communications. High complexity means the contact averages 2 minutes in testing and real-world time. The average internist has about 9,000 emails. The numbers are increasing by 10% a year. It is a huge time-suck. I did the calculation—like 400 hours, just answering questions, whether it's phone calls, med refills, or some query from a patient about some topic.

Another Dean physician said,

> Patient-portal requests through the electronic health record and email are very hot topics right now among primary care physician and nurses. It's more and more what they consider to be non-value-added work being added to their plates.

Thus, virtual medicine may be convenient, but it can also lead to inefficient use of the most valuable part of medicine—the time of physicians, nurse practitioners, and other clinicians. How to triage virtual medicine, to reduce the use of virtual medicine portals by the worried well, better screen incoming communications, train a set of virtual medicine assistants who answer most inquiries, or institute some other technique has not yet been developed. Such triage might look and feel like putting in just the kind of barriers to physician access that virtual medicine was supposed to overcome. Although virtual medicine may enhance patient convenience, it may also exacerbate some types of inefficiency in healthcare. It is certainly not the unalloyed triumph and pivotal element of transformation many techno-utopians avow it to be.

WHY ISN'T VIRTUAL MEDICINE FUNDAMENTAL TO TRANSFORMATION?

The experience of transformed practices and health systems, as well as the existing literature in this area, suggests that virtual medicine is not—at least for the time being—fundamental to the transformation of care delivery. Why?

One reason may be that we do not yet know how to effectively deploy virtual medicine. Proponents of virtual medicine, even if not as insistent as techno-utopians, argue that we must remember that we are still in the early stages. As the technology—and our understanding of how clinicians and patients interact with it—improves, virtual medicine will become more effective at changing health interactions and outcomes. This is the view held by my colleague, Kevin Volpp, the world's leading expert in using behavioral economics to change patient outcomes:

> Right now it is probably true that electronic monitoring and other tech-
> nologies have not been transformative. However, the technology is rap-
> idly evolving in terms of both its capabilities and price. In addition, the
> evidence on how to combine the technology with behavioral solutions
> is also evolving. All of which has the potential to enable significant leaps
> in productivity in managing chronic disease that will not be realizable
> using a personnel-intensive model.

This may, or may not, be right. Regardless, for physicians, nurses, and healthcare leaders who want to transform the delivery of care, this idea means that we are still in the experimental phase of virtual med-icine. The tech-centric future may be far away—if not an impossible future altogether. That means it should not be the focus of transforma-tion today.

Another reason to be skeptical of virtual medicine is the incompati-bility of the target patient population with the technology and the level of knowledge it requires. The high-risk, high-cost patients who need better, high-value care are the Miss Harrises and Mrs. Winstons: chron-ically ill, older adults with limited incomes. These are typically not your tech-savvy innovators, early adopters, or even the early majority. They might use a smartphone and a DVD player, but their interactions with the technological world normally end there. These patients might be willing to use a Web-enabled scale, so long as it is no different from a regular scale and they do not have to remember to charge it or manu-ally link it to something. But any more complicated interactions, such as requiring the patient to regularly look at websites or follow Web in-structions, is unlikely to work. Maybe after 2 or 3 decades, when the current generation of tech-savvy, young adults ages and succumbs to chronic illnesses, wearables and other electronic technologies will be more easily accepted and adopted. However, this is a long time from now. And even this prediction should be skeptically entertained. The dietary study with wearables targeted young adults aged 18 to 35, the tech-savvy demographic. No real impact. There may be something about living with a chronic illness that tends to negate the importance of technological interventions.

A more important barrier to implementation may be the fact that technology is aiming at the wrong end of the loop. The problem is *not* knowing what a chronically ill patient's weight, blood pressure, glucose, or respiratory parameters are at all times but rather what to actually *do* once they are determined to be abnormal. In other words, the barrier is not located in the *sensing*—knowing in real-time that a patient is having a problem—but in *responding* with an effective intervention, one that gets patients to change their behavior while also forestalling additional problems. In short, the real challenge is what biologists and robotics experts call the "effector arm" of healthcare—getting the right interventions to the patient. Technology is great at sensing, and maybe even catergorizing, that information into normal and abnormal. But the key barrier for managing chronic illnesses is not easily or effectively delivered by technology to people. The challenge then is not getting ever more data and information but what to do afterward—which is not necessarily the strong suit of technology companies.

However, there may be an even more important reason why virtual medicine is limited in its impact on clinician-patient interactions: healthcare is fundamentally social. Like all humans, patients respond to people they trust more than robo-calls from a computer or virtual nurses or care coordinators on the phone with whom they have no established relationships. The proper analogy may be how you find interacting with a computerized airline reservation system compared to an actual airline employee. When the problem is serious, like in healthcare, we all prefer personal attention from a real human being.

It is possible to get chronically ill people to change their behavior without the use of virtual medicine. As discussed in Chapters 4 and 6 (pages 95, 96, 137), chronic care managers and behavioral health clinicians can ensure that people with chronic and behavioral health problems stay healthy, while simultaneously ensuring that they go to the ER and hospital less frequently. What the transformed practices in this book show is that, following the identification of at-risk patients, there are 3 key steps to effective interventions: (1) co-location of these providers in physicians' offices; (2) establishment of personal relationships between the care manager, the behavioral health providers, and the patients, which are usually facilitated by physicians; and (3) frequent meetings and personal calls to reinforce the behavioral changes needed. Fundamental to effective change is having a trusted clinician work with the patient. Patients respond to a person they have met and come to trust, one who knows them well and is willing to help create a collaborative strategy with the patient.

Technology can augment the personal relationships between chronic care managers or behavior health clinicians and patients, but only once that relationship has already been established. Technology is not going to replace that relationship—and, honestly, it should not even try. Take, for example, the case of the patients with congestive heart failure whose electronic monitoring technology failed to change their rates of readmission and mortality. We do not precisely understand why the electronic intervention failed, but one possibility is that the intervention lacked the personal touch. When a patient's readings were abnormal, an unknown nurse called the patient and told them to call their healthcare providers. Because the patients did not know or necessarily trust the nurse, they were not incentivized to follow the advice. This is a case in which the technological intervention came between the patient and the care provider.

In successfully transformed practices the approach is different. The chronic care manager, who the patient has known for weeks or months or even years, calls the patient to talk. The patient trusts that the care manager is trying to improve their health. In addition, the care manager has the authority and power to intervene and manage the patient's condition. There is no need for the patient to then initiate another action—calling the physician's office.

THE ROLE OF TECHNOLOGY IN
TRANSFORMED PRACTICES

This does not mean that electronic technology and virtual medicine have no role in transforming care; rather, the main role will not be in replacing the clinician-patient interaction but instead will be in enhancing physicians' diagnostic and management capacities. This will occur in 5 main areas.

First, technology can help physicians manage patients by providing them with real-time, relevant—but not physiological—data. For example, Advocate Health in Chicago was historically plagued by poor readmission rates. In general, Illinois has performed terribly on readmissions. As Lee Sacks, Advocate's CMO put it, "I think Illinois was 48th out of 50 states when they started publishing readmissions data." To counter this, Advocate created a predictive model for readmissions. As he explains,

> We run [the algorithm] in the background on every inpatient. It gets updated every 4 hours based on the clinical situation. It scores people and identifies those at high risk for readmission. It tells the doctor these patients need special attention. And we urge them to have a visit within 48 hours of discharge. The visit doesn't have to be with a physician—it could be a nurse. But with a visit their likelihood of readmission drops immensely.

Technology working in the background can help inpatient management. Yet even then, virtual medicine still requires someone to interact personally with the patient to make it really effective. As Sacks emphasizes,

> Unfortunately, even with this information, our doctors are not clued in to having a visit within 48 hours and don't do it consistently. So we are developing workarounds. We have our home health company and pharmacists visit patients in their home. A lot of the problems that bring patients back in the hospital are medication changes, and pharmacists can help.
>
> Another problem is that even if the physicians tell the patients to call to come into the office for an appointment within 48 hours, the appointments secretary says, "Oh, the next appointment is in 2 weeks." There is just a total disconnect.

Using technology to take scheduling away from physicians' practices, centralizing it, and adding open-access can help address this "total disconnect." In this case, virtual medicine is not about enhancing the clinician-patient interaction; instead, it works in the background, helping physicians overcome the challenges to optimally managing chronically ill patients.

A second area where technology will play a key role is in follow-up for acute care episodes and routine check-ins for relatively stable chronically ill patients. As noted, Iora Health uses text messaging to ensure treatments work for acute but potentially self-limited problems, such as urinary tract infections or minor head trauma. Similarly, Dr. Loftus at Kaiser Permanente Mid-Atlantic hopes to expand the system's use of virtual medicine for follow-up visits. She also thinks that more routine visits—such as checking in every few months with diabetics about their hemoglobin A1c levels, blood pressure, medication adherence, and diet changes—can be done virtually instead of requiring patients to come to the office. It is important to note, however, that in both of these cases the clinician-patient relationships are already well established; the virtual medicine merely supplements the personal interaction. In Dr. Loftus's estimation, virtual follow-ups and routine check-ins *could* reduce physical visits by as much as 40% and would constitute a big savings—lower per capita costs from fewer physical offices, and lower personnel costs from fewer staff doing reception and rooming. But this has yet to be proven.

There are also technological and human challenges to routinely implementing widespread virtual medicine for follow-up and routine care. One deceivingly simple challenge is deciding how to allow physicians to rapidly and seamlessly switch between virtual and in-person visits. There is a natural ebb and flow to physical office visits. If a physician is running a few minutes behind, the receptionist can inform the 1 p.m. patient sitting in the exam room that there will be a 5-minute wait. But a patient with a virtual visit scheduled for 1 p.m. expects it to start promptly at 1 p.m. It is hard to inform them that the physician is running a few minutes late.

A third area in which virtual medicine will transform care is in care for rural patients. No country in the world has really solved the problem of providing excellent care to rural patients. Well-educated physicians and other clinicians prefer to live in larger metropolitan or suburban areas thriving with cultural attractions, diversity, and social events. Numerous attempts to induce physicians to locate in rural areas, whether through incentives or penalties, have failed almost everywhere they have been tried. Virtual medicine that allows physicians to live where they want but treat patients who live in rural areas may finally solve the drought of physicians in these areas. Nurses could be the primary care providers in rural areas, with physicians available virtually for more complex cases or emergencies. In this situation physicians, even primary care physicians, would serve more like consultants with periodic assessments who support the primary care nurses.

Another function of virtual medicine might be to facilitate physician-to-physician consultations. Many specialist physicians, such as dermatologists, pediatric specialists, and psychiatrists, are in short supply. Virtual medicine might allow physicians to obtain real-time consultations from these specialists. At Kaiser Permanente, using cell phone cameras has dramatically increased the number of dermatology consultations a dermatologist can perform while in his or her office. Again, this augments care not by supplanting the physician-patient relationship but by offering timely assistance to the patient's physician.

Another area where virtual medicine will come into play is when machine learning allows computers to replace physicians. Machine learning can break into the field of medicine by utilizing huge digital datasets. Computers will learn from the billions of existing digital radiographs and pathology slides and can then apply the learned skills in identifying tumors and other abnormalities. Within the next decade machines will largely replace diagnostic radiologists and anatomical pathologists. The machine learning aspect of virtual medicine will then replace anesthesiologists and critical care physicians who monitor a relatively small number of physiological indicators and adjust medications and other interventions in response to abnormalities. Machines will learn how to expertly manage anesthetized and critically ill patients better than tired physicians.

Before machine learning can displace critical care physicians, virtual medicine will first optimize care of critically ill patients through tele-ICUs. During the night shift at Banner Hospitals in Phoenix, all of the sites are equipped with tele-ICU, which links patients to intensive care physicians in locations where it is daytime, such as Tel-Aviv, Israel. The physicians have a camera trained on the patients, as well as real-time data feeds with the patients' medications and physiological data—heart rate and rhythm, blood pressure, oxygenation, fluid balances, and other physiological indicators. If something unexpected happens, these remote physicians can see the abnormal data, check on the patient, talk to the nurses, and manage the patient remotely. And these physicians can do so during daytime—at least for them—while they are wide awake. One virtual physician also has the ability to monitor scores of patients. Tele-ICU has been in place at Banner since 2006. It has taken time to fully integrate into patient care, but after the initial learning curve, the results have been impressive. In 2013, for instance, its tele-ICU saved 33,000 ICU days and $89 million. Not surprisingly, Banner has continued to expand the program.

AS SHOWN BY PLACES like Kaiser Permanente, Iora Health, and Banner, we are now in the very earliest days of a virtual medicine boom. But for all the fanfare that currently surrounds this field, it still plays a rather limited role in actually providing care to those patients outside the system and without trusted primary care providers. However, virtual medicine has proven successful in optimizing care for those patients already established in the system, though its role is by no means transformative.

Virtual medicine may be helpful, but is not fundamental to transformation. Its impact is largely dependent upon the presence of a clinician's human touch, which may be better informed by the technology—but technology cannot replace high touch care. For now human interaction remains the lynchpin of the effectively transformed office or health system. Maybe, after experimentation and optimization, virtual medicine will turn out to be capable of radically transforming care delivery. But that means it cannot be the focus of a practice or health system's transformation in the next decade. Indeed, I am skeptical that it will ever replace the clinician-patient relationship.

Chapter 8

IS TRANSFORMED
HEALTHCARE
TRANSFERABLE?

IS ALL HEALTHCARE LOCAL?

Historically, many health policy experts have expressed skepticism regarding the feasibility of transferring high-value delivery system reforms to a new geographic location. This wariness is not baseless—many groups have failed to scale their models. Ironically, a prime example of this failure is Kaiser Permanente.

By integrating insurance with healthcare delivery, Kaiser Permanente assumes full financial risk in order to provide organizational-level incentives to keep costs down. Front-line physicians are paid salaries with bonuses for providing high-quality care, unlike the traditional fee-for-service model that incentivizes higher volumes and higher costs. Kaiser's payment model works: by numerous objective assessments Kaiser Permanente does achieve consistently high-value care. Its Medicare Advantage plans in northern and southern California are both Medicare 5-star plans and are often placed first—or at least in the top 10 nationally—in *U.S. News and World Report*, *Consumer Reports*, and various other rankings. Kaiser's successes are further bolstered by the fact that its premiums are relatively low. While they are said to "shadow price"—slightly undercut premiums of—Blue Cross and Blue Shield plans, they still represent lower cost even if not as low as some might think possible. Consequently, numerous health policy experts have argued that expanding Kaiser Permanente everywhere in the United States would be a step in the right direction, improving the nation's healthcare, while simultaneously lowering costs.

Attempts to transfer the Kaiser model, however, have largely been dismal failures. Kaiser started in the late 1930s and early 1940s at the Grand Coulee Dam construction site in Washington State and the Richmond shipyards in Oakland, California. With the end of World War II came a drop in employment at the construction sites and ship-yards; enrollment in Kaiser Permanente likewise declined. In response, Kaiser opened enrollment to the public. Many workers already knew of and liked Kaiser, so enrolling them, given that Kaiser had established administrative and delivery systems, was easy. Kaiser quickly saw their membership rates surge once again.

Over the years, Kaiser has been very successful in California and Or-egon. Yet expansion beyond these traditional geographic regions has repeatedly flopped, despite favorable dynamics, such as the enactment of the Health Maintenance Organization (HMO) Act of 1973 that re-quired employers with over 25 employees who offer health insurance to offer the option of a federally certified HMO. Kaiser outposts in Texas, North Carolina, Ohio, and the Northeast all failed and were then sold, spun off, or closed. Attempts by Kaiser to expand into Georgia, Col-orado, and the DC-Maryland-Virginia area, although not so bad that operations had to be closed or sold off, have struggled. After 70 years of being open to the public, lauded by policy experts, and supported by federal legislation, Kaiser provides care to just over 10 million Ameri-cans, of whom 82% are in the original states of California and Oregon. Thus, Kaiser itself seems to be the prime example of proving that trans-ferring a better model that delivers high-value care into new healthcare ecosystems is virtually impossible.

Why is there a transferability problem at all? In the view of some leading health policy experts, the answer is that "all healthcare is lo-cal." In an article entitled "Fail to Scale," health policy experts Jeff Goldsmith and Lawton Burns (a colleague of mine at the University of Pennsylvania's Wharton School) argue that Kaiser is simply the pro-totypical case of an inherent problem in trying to expand healthcare models into new geographies. Drawing on the analogy of terroir in wine, Goldsmith and Burns claim that there are unique local historical, cultural, political, and economic factors that "color the traditions of medical practice and health care organization" in different communi-ties, and that these local factors preclude solutions to the problems that plague the American healthcare system. In Kaiser Permanente's case, 3 factors unique to the Oregon and California markets made it possible for its model of care to grow: "large multispecialty group practice[s], a tradition of prepayment for health services (as opposed to indemnity insurance), and large unionized employers." Kaiser Permanente's large presence in West Coast markets made the switch from unionized construction and shipyard workers to the public easy because of brand recognition and low sales costs. These factors never existed in other geographic regions.

Goldsmith and Burns point out that Kaiser Permanente's story is not unique. Other attempts to expand successful healthcare organizations outside of their home turf have failed. The recent attempts by what originally was a dialysis company, DeVita, to spread HealthCare Partners, a successful southern California primary care organization, have "struggled to achieve either market influence or profitability." Goldsmith and Burns argue that "there seems to be almost nothing except Medicare that is truly national about our health system. Fort Lauderdale, FL, Hastings, NE, and Seattle, WA, are actually in different countries culturally and politically." Thus, attempts to apply "single bullet policy solutions . . . have resulted in a lengthening string of policy disappointments." According to Goldsmith and Burns, the terroir effect means there is little chance of replicating successfully transformed physician practices or health systems in different regions of the country. Ultimately each transformed practice or system needs to grow up in its particular locality and healthcare ecosystem—successful healthcare organizations cannot be imported from another region of the country.

It is important to note that the real challenge of transformation is not what Silicon Valley types usually call "scalability." Few doubt the ability of one physician practice, multispecialty group, or health system to grow in its local area. After all, Dean Clinic grew from a small system to cover 22 counties in southern Wisconsin. WESTMED in Westchester County, New York, grew from 14 physicians in the late 1980s to nearly 350 physicians today. CareMore grew from a few offices in Los Angeles in 1991 to serving approximately 80,000 patients across southern California today. The challenge for transformation in healthcare delivery, therefore, is less *scalability* and more *transferability*. Can a physician practice, multispecialty group, or a health system that delivers higher-quality and lower-cost care repeat its achievement in a distinct geographic location with different cultural, social, economic, and other histories and medical practices?

If Goldsmith and Burns are correct and it is indeed impossible to transfer transformed delivery systems, then this book is worthless. If all healthcare is local and the specific healthcare ecosystem of a city or state shapes what changes are possible, then describing what happens in Westchester, New York; Chicago, Illinois; Madison, Wisconsin; or Orange County, California, is unhelpful to physicians and health managers who want to transform their practices in, say, Grand Rapids, Michigan, or Birmingham, Alabama. According to Goldsmith and Burns different communities will need different transformation strategies. The particular financial, physician, hospital, and other arrangements that make Advocate Health Care able to deliver high-value care in the metropolitan Chicago area are not available to the 29-physician Southview Medical Group in Birmingham. Similarly, Madison is not Atlanta. The knowledge CareMore accrued with Medicare patients in southern California would not help if it wanted to improve care for Medicaid patients in Des Moines, Iowa, with a totally different set of hospitals, physicians, durable medical equipment suppliers, and home-care agencies. Similarly, VillageMD's experience in Houston would not help it transform primary care in Bloomington.

However, experts like Goldsmith and Burns who argue that delivery system innovations are not transferable are making critical mistakes. Goldsmith and Burns claim that the organizational structure of a system like Kaiser Permanente or Dean Clinic cannot be transferred. Although this may or may not be true, this argument is ultimately irrelevant. What needs to be transferred for successful transformation is not an entire organizational structure, but rather the 12 transformational practices delineated in Chapters 4 through 6. A physician group does not have to emulate everything done by VillageMD, an oncology group does not have to become a clone of Main Line Oncology, a multispecialty group does not have to become WESTMED, and a health system does not have to become Kaiser Permanente to provide high-quality, lower-cost care—it simply needs to adopt the transformational practices of a successful system in a tiered approach. Although implementing the 12 transformational practices may not be easy—some practices might do it poorly and even fail—and will require significant leadership, data, and payment changes, possibly in response to an existential crisis, it is nevertheless much easier than trying to recreate the entire organizational apparatus of a CareMore or an Advocate Health Care.

Although healthcare may be local and healthcare organizational structures may be geographically constrained based on history, state laws, the structure of the local hospital markets, and local financial arrangements, transformational practices are generalizable. In this sense, the processes of care can be transformed and exist in any number of different delivery structures—smaller primary care or specialty physician groups, multispecialty groups, specialty groups, and larger health systems. Structure and process do not have to be tightly coupled. These transformational practices can be replicated in new healthcare ecosystems. Ultimately, adopting at least a subset of these 12 practices will allow physician groups and systems to deliver consistently higher-quality and more cost-effective care to patients. The proper question, therefore, is not whether all healthcare is truly local, but rather: Can physician practices, multispecialty groups, and health systems adopt a core group of transformational practices to consistently deliver high-value care?

Ultimately, the answer is yes. Any organization committed to transforming themselves to provide higher-value care can adopt the 12 practices, regardless of their geographic location, state laws, or local history. Although there are foundational management and financial elements that must be in place prior to implementing any of these practices (see Chapters 2 and 3), the process of transformation is possible in essentially any health marketplace within the United States—and maybe beyond. The 12 practices can be found in almost every corner of the country—and with them, the chance at true transformation.

EXAMPLES OF THE TRANSFERABILITY OF TRANSFORMED PRACTICES

Goldsmith and Burns cite Kaiser Permanente as the quintessential example of the "failure to scale" and use it to generalize about the impossibility of transferring transformations to high-value care. Yet Kaiser could just as easily be used as an example of the opposite—the possibility of transferring transformed medical organizations.

Kaiser Mid-Atlantic is 2,800 miles away from the "original" Kaiser Permanente on the West Coast. The Washington, DC–Maryland-Virginia region is certainly in a distinct terroir—no one would mistake Virginian wines for Napa or Willamette Valley offerings. And the Washington area is heavily dependent on the federal government for employment which is not true of California and Oregon. In the 2000s Kaiser Mid-Atlantic was failing, seeming to confirm the claim that all medicine is local. But was this failure, as Goldsmith and Burns would have it, inherently due to the terroir effect—the different cultural, structural, and financial history of the mid-Atlantic region? Or was it attributable to flawed management that failed to effectively implement the best Kaiser Permanente practices that deliver high-value care?

No one transplanted new "earth and vines"—the medical culture of multispecialty groups, capitation, and unionized employers found in northern California and Oregon—in 2009 to replicate the Kaiser terroir in Washington, DC, Virginia, and Maryland. And yet since 2009, Kaiser Permanente Mid-Atlantic has managed to transform itself to deliver high-value care. How? By bringing in better management and implementing key transformational practices. Over the past 8 years, Kaiser Permanente Mid-Atlantic has become the best health system in not only its region but also among the very best in the nation for all measures, including quality, access, patient experience, and cost. The National Committee for Quality Assurance (NCQA) awarded Kaiser Mid-Atlantic its top ranking, 5.0, for private health insurance plans in the country. Only 13 private health insurance plans, out of 1,000 included by the NCQA, received a 5.0 ranking. On many specific measures, Kaiser is also a regional and national leader. It is number 1 in the region and in the top quartile nationally for blood pressure control. Kaiser's achievements in blood pressure control encompass not only white patients but also patients of all races and ethnicities. High-quality outcomes have come with significant cost reductions too. Since 2009 Kaiser Permanente Mid-Atlantic has reduced emergency room use per thousand members by 20% and inpatient hospital days per thousand members by 24%. This success in quality and cost has translated into significant membership growth. In 2008 and 2009, about 470,000 people were enrolled in Kaiser Mid-Atlantic. By 2016 membership had increased by nearly 40% to over 650,000.

How did Kaiser Permanente Mid-Atlantic transform itself? There were 5 major steps. First, it dramatically improved its scheduling. Upon hiring more primary care physicians and establishing new clinical decision units that served as full-service urgent-care centers, Kaiser Permanente was able to expand from a 9 to 5 operation to a 24/7 system. By doing so it decreased patient waiting times for appointments and also allowed physicians to spend more time with seriously ill patients. Kaiser Permanente patients now wait an average of 6 days for a dermatology appointment, compared to the average 15-day wait at outside systems.

Second, Kaiser modified their rooming practices by creating a system in which every caregiver is responsible for closing care gaps. At every visit in every part of Kaiser Permanente, the EHR automatically brings up patients' care gaps. If a patient seen in the ophthalmology clinic needs a mammogram, the staff in the ophthalmologist's office are alerted and entrusted with scheduling it.

Third, Kaiser focused on improving care management of high-risk, high-cost patients. It created health tools such as disease registries and "on-demand" searches for patients' full data to identify high-risk patients. Kaiser then entrusted the primary care teams to reach out to these patients and bring them into their network. This care management is not outsourced but instead "owned by the primary care team, not a third party."

Fourth, Kaiser instituted rigorous performance measurement. Physicians are measured on quality-of-care metrics, and the results are released in an identifiable manner. Thus, there are physician-by-physician comparative results on quality metrics, such as percent of diabetic patients with hemoglobin A1c over 9.0%. This ensures transparency and also allows clinicians who may not be performing at the top to find out what the successful clinicians are doing to excel so they can then emulate their practices.

Finally, Kaiser developed a strategy related to the hospitals and other facilities it contracts with to improve care and lower costs, especially hospital costs. It established 5 large Hubs—full service ambulatory and urgent care facilities with imaging, laboratory, medical, and surgical services to substitute for sending patients to urgent care or emergency rooms (see page 165). It also negotiated better hospital contracts, concentrating its hospitalized patients in 10 high-performing facilities out of the regions' more than 32 hospitals.

The transformation of Kaiser Permanente Mid-Atlantic—namely, its turnaround from nearly closing in 2009 to becoming one of the nation's highest-performing health systems on quality, cost, and patient satisfaction—casts doubt on the validity of the terroir effect. It indicates that the impossibility of transferring the transformational practices is overstated. What we need to focus on is not transferring organizations and their structures but transferring transformational processes and practices.

Furthermore, Kaiser Permanente Mid-Atlantic is not the only example of successfully transferring transformational practices. For instance, CareMore is trying to move into the Medicaid markets in Memphis and Des Moines, and is currently working with Emory in Atlanta—all markets outside of CareMore's southern California home base. Its expansion process has not been without challenges. Its signature is high-touch, low-cost, high-access care. Two of CareMore's key practices are the use of chronic care managers and rapidly shifting care out of the hospital to lower cost facilities or home. The extensivist and care-manager program rapidly shifts patients from hospital to home with extensive home care services. Executing that requires careful coordination with home-care and durable medical equipment companies to ensure the oxygen, hospital beds, portable commodes, and other equipment are in the home when the patient arrives and, as the CEO says, "the home care nurses are showing up and are doing what they need to be doing." Attention to the myriad "minor details is critical to making a new site successful." And this cannot be underestimated. But how CareMore succeeded was by *not* aiming to replicate its southern California organizational structure, but rather by implementing its proven processes of care.

In Memphis, CareMore faced 2 key challenges: focusing more chronic care management resources on chronically ill patients and changing scheduling and site of service to ensure the Medicaid population stopped going to the emergency room for routine care. As CareMore CEO Sachin Jain explains:

We have done things like extend hours, so now our offices are open 7 a.m. to 7 p.m. It is a nurse-practitioner-based primary care system with long visits. We have also implemented an ER avoidance program to try to get them to use CareMore offices before going to the ER.

Some patients had diabetes for 7 years but didn't really know it because they had been told to take a pill without really understanding what the pill was for. So we take the time to educate them about their disease and develop a care plan around the patient.

It is too early to tell if CareMore will succeed in transforming care in Memphis and Des Moines. Regardless, it is important to note that CareMore is approaching the new locales not by trying to replicate its organizational structure but rather by replicating its most successful practices—extended schedules, chronic care management, and changing the site of service out of the hospital to the home.

Others are trying to transfer their practices too. ChenMed has begun successfully transforming practices in Richmond, Virginia; Louisville, Kentucky; and other places. WESTMED is trying to replicate its model with a Medicaid population in Brooklyn, New York. VillageMD has expanded to Indianapolis, New Hampshire, and Chicago, with other markets in the planning phases.

A TIERED TRANSFORMATIONAL PROCESS

No physician office, multispecialty group, or even larger health system can implement all 12 transformational practices at once. No organization can have that broad a bandwidth and stand that much disruption. Indeed, I have yet to find any single organization, no matter how long they have been working on delivery system transformation, doing all 12 practices. For instance, CareMore has been on its transformation journey for decades, yet open-access scheduling is not routine. WESTMED has limited use of shared decision making. Kaiser Permanente Mid-Atlantic has just begun to introduce its own version of CareMore's extensivist as a model of care management for its sickest patients. Aledade focused first on scheduling, performance measurement, and chronic care management but not site of service and palliative care.

Offices, groups, and health systems embarking on transformation must prioritize what steps should be undertaken first, and which ones can be delayed to the second and third tiers of implementation. The prioritization decisions should be influenced by characteristics of a practice or group's specific patient population, the nature of contracts with payers, the amount of financial gain for improving quality versus reducing total cost of care, and other technical issues. Nevertheless, some general guidance about how to tier transformation is possible.

Of the 12 practices, the 4 highest-priority ones—tier-1 transformational practices—are scheduling, performance measurement, chronic-care coordination, and site of service (see Table 8.1, page 233). Any physician office or medical group can extend office hours and implement open-access scheduling. These practices are relatively easy to implement, and there is reasonably good guidance already available on the technical aspects. More importantly, these practices greatly enhance patient satisfaction and access to care. They will improve office efficiency by reducing no-shows, and decrease patient utilization of more expensive services such as visits to the emergency room. Indeed, probably more than any change, it is simply important to demonstrate to patients that a medical group is committed to being patient-centric.

Performance measurement is another critical initial practice. It is hard for physicians and care teams to improve their care delivery if they have no idea how well or poorly they are actually performing relative to objective standards. Because Medicare and many contracts with private insurance companies financially reward high quality and/or improving quality, providing feedback to physicians and care teams about their performance is key to reducing unnecessary services, ensuring care gaps are closed, and improving financial results.

If there is one necessary transformation, it is chronic care coordination. Because 84% of healthcare spending in the United States is for chronic illness, having dedicated chronic care coordinators embedded within the primary care teams—and even specialist physicians' offices, such as oncologists' and cardiologists' offices—ensures that patients understand their illness, comply with medications and other prescribed interventions, and call the office rather than use the emergency room. Therefore, chronic care coordinators are one of the best ways to improve quality and reduce costs. Chronic care coordinators can also be highly effective in ensuring smooth transitions of care and that pa-tients recently discharged from the hospital or skilled nursing facility (SNF) are contacted by a nurse practitioner or primary care physician within 48 hours or, at most a week, to reduce readmissions.

If the findings of this book suggest anything, it is that no group needs to reinvent the wheel. Multiple physician groups, multigroup practices, and health systems have successfully implemented the same basic model of effective chronic care coordination, following the same 5 steps (see pages 97–99) in many different geographic locations.

The final tier-1 transformational practice is one that is often over-looked: site of service. Some accountable care organizations (ACOs), like Aledade, have found that primary care physicians can do all the right things—reduce emergency room use, hospitalizations, and re-admissions by 5%—and still lose because of referrals and site-of-service costs. We know the prices of physicians and facilities vary tremendously; so too do physicians' proclivities to order unnecessary tests and treat-ments. According to one of its senior executives, when Blue Cross Blue Shield of Massachusetts ran its Alternative Quality Contract program,

> More than half of the savings was associated with changing site of ser-vice, meaning using lower-cost settings. There was no change in the amount of care, but a change in price by delivering the care somewhere different.
>
> In the very early days, this change in the site of care focused on kinds of care where there are no relationships at stake, like lab tests and imag-ing and colonoscopies where as long as it is a convenient location the patient doesn't particularly care where they go.
>
> Later it did involve changing hospitals and specialists to ones that had lower prices.

The 2nd tier of transformation should focus on registration and rooming, standardization of care, de-institutionalization, and behav-ioral health. This recommendation is conditional. Registration and rooming is another one of those largely ignored steps of transforma-tion, but when done well can be both effective and efficient. It can pro-vide a structured mechanism to automate a labor-intensive process and to use otherwise "wasted" time during an office visit to ensure all gaps in care are closed. Registration can be effectively automated by systems like those deployed at ChenMed and Certify, thereby reducing fraud and duplicate records as well as redeploying front office personnel to more valuable activities. Similarly, the responsibility for rooming should be entrusted to a medical assistant empowered with information about the care gaps and authority to order tests, immunizations, and treatments. Giving these tasks, often considered annoying by physicians, to other care providers can be a win-win-win—increasing the quality of care, reducing physician dissatisfaction, and increasing medical assistant job satisfaction. Because there is usually some financial reward from payers for closing care gaps, the higher quality and efficiency can simultaneously increase revenue.

The good thing about standardization of care—also part of the 2nd-tier practices—is that there are many useful guidelines, pathways, and protocols readily available that can be adopted in patient care. What makes standardization difficult—and why it is in the 2nd tier—is deciding how to integrate these pathways and protocols into the electronic health record so they show up as standing order sets. Yet once accomplished, standardization can help improve physician and staff efficiency and reduce both unjustifiable variation in care and the number of unnecessary tests and treatments. It also provides more agreed-upon metrics for performance measurement.

De-institutionalization, namely moving patients out of the hospital, rehabilitation, and other facilities and into care at home, is generally also in the 2nd tier. A significant amount of de-institutionalization will be achieved indirectly by preempting hospitalizations through chronic care management and reducing readmissions. More direct de-institutionalization depends upon having good contracts with reliable and high-quality home-care agencies, durable medical equipment suppliers, and excellent palliative- and hospice-care providers. If full de-institutionalization cannot be achieved, some practices and systems can at least decrease the costs of institutional care by rapidly shifting patients from expensive hospitals to lower-cost skilled nursing facilities (SNFs) Because transformed medical groups and health systems usually have their own hospitalists caring for patients within the SNF, they are able to ensure higher-quality care. Preliminary evidence for the financial benefits of de-institutionalization comes from the ACO examples, where physician-led ACOs did better in terms of saving money than hospital-led ACOs.

One of the bigger challenges of transformation is behavioral and mental health. After care coordination for chronic illnesses, improving behavioral and mental healthcare for patients with depression, anxiety, and substance abuse disorders probably represents a big opportunity for quality improvement and cost savings. Recently physician practices and health systems that have been on the transformation journey for years have begun to experiment with different approaches to addressing behavioral health. They are in the early phases of figuring out the best models. The specific details of the most efficient practices are not yet clear but will likely be some version of the collaborative care model that can be deployed in primary and specialty practices. It remains to be determined whether this will be similar to the Advocate and Central Medical Clinic model of co-locating behavioral health specialists in the physician office or a more virtual approach like that promulgated by Quartet (see pages 140–141). Regardless, the next decade will illuminate the advantages and challenges of implementing behavioral health interventions, especially for depression, anxiety, and substance abuse, and will offer transforming organizations more proven models to choose from.

The 3rd tier of transformation involves practices that, in general, have been adopted by fewer transformed organizations and still need refining. Although most patient populations need lifestyle interventions, the return is more long term. However, if a physician practice or group has a very high proportion of the frail elderly, for whom falls and the subsequent need for hip replacements are of serious concern, interventions that focus on improving patients' balance and strength may provide rapid return. Although some larger health systems may emulate CareMore's lead and invest in a network of their own exercise facilities, smaller physician groups and practices may simply contract with local YMCAs, gyms, and others to offer free tai chi, yoga and other exercise classes to patients. However, lifestyle interventions are likely to be a lower priority for many providers on the path to transformation.

Shared decision making is another 3rd-tier transformation practice. Luckily, many decision aides, covering hundreds of interventions, are readily available from several companies. Yet having decision aides is necessary but not sufficient. Staff must be able to work with patients to access and view the decision aides. The aides should be consistently integrated into care workflows in order to ensure that physicians and other members of the care team are comfortable discussing the material. For some physicians, especially those with older patients who have a high rate of hip and knee replacements, shared decision making may be of higher priority. Otherwise, the return in terms of quality, patient satisfaction with care decisions, and cost savings are likely to put this important step in transformation further down on the priority list.

These are broad guidelines on how to tier transformational practices; they will need modifications for different types of practices. For orthopedic or cardiothoracic surgeons under bundles, de-institutionalization and shifting patients out of SNFs and rehabilitation facilities to home care may be a higher priority, as it is central to cost savings. Similarly, for oncologists and others clinicians who deal with advanced and terminally ill patients, end-of-life care may be the most pressing problem. For these specialists, having a high-quality palliative care provider like Aspire readily available may be a high priority. For physician groups or organizations with a high proportion of low-income, socially stressed patients, effective community healthcare workers may become a tier-1 practice.

Instituting some of these transformational practices must be done by the medical organization itself. Changing rooming guidelines, or co-locating chronic care coordinators in the practice, are steps that cannot be outsourced. Indeed, part of the success of the practice depends upon the personnel in the medical organization "owning" the practice. Others can be outsourced. For instance, there exist companies that can partner and provide effective approaches to registration, palliative care, and maybe even behavioral and mental healthcare. Contracting with these companies may make it easier to change certain practices and speed up the transformation.

THE TIMING OF TRANSFORMATION

How long should it take to transform a physician practice, multispecialty group, or health system? Many commentators wait only 1 or 2 years after an organization begins transforming before deciding whether the effort has been a failure. For instance, the ACO initiative has been widely criticized because after a few years it has saved only a few hundred million dollars. Critics also point to the Oregon experiment, in which low-income people were enrolled in Medicaid yet showed no significant improvement in blood pressure, cholesterol, or diabetes 2 years later. When commentators see these types of short-term results, they declare the experiments in transformation to be failures.

Transformation does not happen overnight. It takes time—and more time than many understandably impatient people in healthcare seem willing to wait. When Blue Cross Blue Shield of Massachusetts embarked on its Alternative Quality Contracts (AQC), they allotted 5 years to the program, longer than the usual 3-year contracts. As the senior executives argued, physician practices needed a longer time horizon to invest in infrastructure, learn how to change their practices, and make multiple refinements to the changes. And these senior executives were right. The data indicate that the improvement happened in the first year, but it was not until the fourth year that the entire AQC arrangement actually began reducing overall costs.

Similarly, data from Medicare's ACOs suggest that those sticking with the program are improving their performance as time progresses. They are learning what works and changing their practices. But this takes time. As Farzad Mostashari, CEO of Aledade, wrote in an article,

> An increasing proportion of ACOs have generated savings above their minimum savings rate each year, and success appears to increase with the number of years in the [ACO] program: increasing from 21% of first year ACOs to 42% of ACOs that were in their fourth year.

At Kaiser Permanente Mid-Atlantic, transformation took about 6 years. In 2006, the plan was ranked number 133 in the nation by NCQA; by 2012 it had risen to number 15, and by 2016 it was ranked in the top tier of the entire country along with only 12 other health plans. At Dean Clinic they were doing so poorly that they had "a burning platform during 2005 and 2006." They initiated their transformation in response. Over the course of 6 years Dean rose to be the top-ranked healthcare system in their region. Similarly, John Sprandio's transformation of his oncology practice took time. His practice first put into place their own EHR, then began standardizing care pathways and measuring their performance, and finally created an algorithm-driven call center to manage chemotherapy side effects and other problems. After 4 years, emergency room use dropped by 50%; after 7 years, it had dropped by nearly 70%.

Others, such as Iora Health and VillageMD, have started "fresh," creating their own primary care clinics and hiring their own physicians. In these cases there was no crisis that catalyzed change; instead, these groups tried to create a transformed delivery system from day 1.

Expecting a transformation to take 5 to 7 years in healthcare is in line with transformation timelines in other business domains. John Kotter, a world leading business theorist on change, argues that change actually takes a long time. In his famous article, "Leading Change: Why Transformation Efforts Fail," Kotter claims,

> Renewal takes not months but years. . . . After a few years of hard work, managers may be tempted to declare victory with the first clear performance improvement. While celebrating a win is fine, declaring the war won can be catastrophic.

When his team quantified the amount of change that occurred each year at transformed companies, the maximum amount of change was found to occur during the 5th year of transformation. Overall, Kotter argues that for transformation to really take hold within an organization, that group must be willing to wait somewhere between 5 to 10 years. Until the changes are firmly implemented, "new approaches are fragile and subject to regression."

Understanding this time frame is critical. First, it preempts both premature memorial services for failed transformations and premature victory celebrations after a few successful improvements. The vocal damnation of ACOs as failed after just a few years seems premature, as does the negative assessments of the impact of Oregon's Medicaid experiment on patients' health outcomes. Second, recognizing that transformation requires at least 5 years reminds us that we need to be modest about what to expect after only a few years; for example, it is unlikely that people can change their care-seeking behaviors in just one year. Third, understanding this time frame can help minimize the chances of failure because it gives people more realistic expectations. In 1 to 3 years, reducing the use of the emergency room by 5% or the re-admission rate by 10% are realistic goals. Achieving them keeps people marching in the direction of transformation and not giving up. In this way, realistic expectations allow for the sustained effort over 5 years, necessary for deep transformation. Fourth, knowing this timeline also helps create the proper types of contracts between payers and provid-ers. These contracts can include intermediate performance targets, but a 5-year contract for transformation is more realistic than a 3-year one. The change in the contract length instituted by Blue Cross Blue Shield of Massachusetts is an excellent model. It also suggests that Medicare needs to change from 3-year contracts to 5-year contracts on its ACO, bundled payment, and other alternative-payment models.

TRANSFORMATION OF healthcare is an ongoing process, not a one-time event. Transforming physician practices, multispecialty groups, and health systems is hard work that takes time. There is a great deal of skepticism that it is possible. This book argues that transformation is not about instituting one or even a few organizational models through-out the entire country. Instead, transformation is about implementing the transformational practices that are transferable from medical orga-nization to medical organization in different regions. These transfor-mational practices are moveable and adoptable. I have found the same basic practices of scheduling, performance measurement, chronic care coordination, and site of service in very different organizations located in very different communities throughout the country.

No organization can institute all 12 transformational practices all at once. No organization has the management capacity to do that. They are best phased in through a deliberate, 3-tiered process. This phasing-in takes time to be fully incorporated into an organization's culture—up to 10 years. The healthcare community should be realis-tic about this timeframe in order to properly set expectations among healthcare workers and commentators as well as to negotiate contracts.

Because transformation is difficult and takes time, I have tried to give realistic timelines. By 2020 or so most medical organizations could use open-access scheduling, the basic elements of performance measurement, and chronic care coordination. These practices have been developed and are already operational in many different physician practices, multispecialty groups, and health systems today. It will take longer, perhaps until 2025 or so, for many organizations to institute other critical practices such as behavioral health interventions, which are still in the experimental stage and need refinement. Nevertheless, it is clear that the process of transformation can start now and will evolve over the next 10 to 15 years.

By 2030, healthcare in the United States should be much better than it is today.

Chapter 9

HOW TO PICK
YOUR DOCTOR

"ZEKE, I NEED A DOCTOR. Who should I go to?"

I am frequently asked this question. An acquaintance wants me to recommend a primary care physician. The relative of a family friend has just been diagnosed with cancer and wants "the best." Even my daughter who has moved to a new city wants me to find her an obstetrician-gynecologist. What do I do? Honestly, in the end I am not very methodical or rigorous about it. I refer them to physicians I trained with in residency and a fellowship program, to former colleagues, or, as I recently did for my daughter, I will call a colleague I trust in the new city and ask for their recommendation.

For many people without a physician friend they can call, their information often comes from the "top doctors" listings in magazines. Yet their methodologies are not very rigorous. Most magazines base their rankings on reputation among other physicians or borrow a ranking that is not based on any objective performance assessment. The *Washingtonian,* for example, surveys local physicians and asks them to name the doctors they would send a family member to in each of 40 specialties. Usually over 1,000 physicians reply to this survey. The physicians with the most votes are named "top doctors." *Philadelphia Magazine* relies on Castle Connolly Medical, which solicits nominations and then lets a "physician-led research team" choose. But there is no suggestion that these teams use any standardized performance data.

QUESTIONS TO ASK A POTENTIAL PHYSICIAN

Is there a better way? I believe there is. The 12 transformational practices provide a framework for determining whether potential physician
practices have changed to be more patient-centric and provide consistently high-quality, lower-cost care (see Table 9.1, page 234).

In seeking out a physician, there are 2 absolutely necessary practices
to focus on and ask questions about (see Table 9.2, page 235). The first is
open-access scheduling. You want a physician office, whether primary
care or specialty, where you can be seen the same day if you are sick
or are having a complication from care you received or drug you are
taking. You do not want to wait days or weeks for the next available
physician appointment. Having open-access scheduling is probably
the clearest way a physician office or group can communicate that they
take their patients' time and discomfort seriously. Open-access scheduling means the practice is organized around patient convenience
rather than physician preferences. If the practice or group does not
have open-access scheduling, I would think hard about whether you
want to be their patient.

The second absolutely necessary practice is performance measurement. As a patient you want a top-quality practice, one that is committed to constantly improving the quality of its care. The only way
a practice can improve—and know it is improving—is by measuring
how well it is doing and by comparing its performance to national
benchmarks. How can you tell whether a practice or group is engaged
in systematic performance measurement? One reliable way is to determine whether the practice is recognized by the National Committee
for Quality Assurance (NCQA) as a Patient Centered Medical Home
(PCMH), essentially the argot of the field.

NCQA is a private, not-for-profit organization committed to performance assessment. Their process for recognizing PCMHs began over a
decade ago and has since evolved. For 2017, NCQA has issued another
revision of their standards and processes that strongly emphasizes patient centeredness and patient outcomes. For patients, the important
point is that the NCQA process emphasizes the "collection of performance data and analysis, setting goals and acting to improve practice
performance, and sharing practice performance data and analysis." In

particular, the assessment focuses on reporting and improving across 35 quality performance indicators, including for children, immunizations and appropriate treatment of upper respiratory infections; and for adults, preventive care such as mammograms, Pap smears, colonoscopies, appropriate use of imaging for lower-back pain, controlling high blood pressure, and appropriate medications for heart failure. PCMH recognition also emphasizes same-day routine and urgent-care appointments (scheduling transformation) as well as more integrated behavioral and mental healthcare, including screening with a standardized questionnaire for depression and anxiety and someone who can coordinate patients' behavioral health needs (behavioral health transformation).

From a patient's perspective, I think the details of the actual NCQA assessment of physician practices are less important than whether those practices have initiated the NCQA process, thereby explicitly signaling their dedication not only to performance measurement but also to improvement.

Physician practices that have open-access scheduling and participate in performance measurement through NCQA PCMH recognition are committed to delivering high-quality, patient-focused care. This is the baseline threshold for selecting a primary care physician for the majority of Americans who have relatively minor health problems and no significant chronic health conditions.

Even for these relatively healthy Americans, it would be highly desirable—although not absolutely necessary—to select practices that have begun to standardize care. A pediatric practice should have adopted a standard care pathway or protocol for evaluating and treating upper-respiratory infections, ear infections, and asthma. Similarly, it would be desirable for an internal medicine practice to have standardized their care for managing high blood pressure, high cholesterol, migraines, and lower-back pain. Asking whether the practice has standardized pathways or protocols for common conditions—and if the answer is yes, what types of conditions—is simple and nonoffensive. Patients are unlikely to inquire about the details of the protocol. What is important is the fact that the physicians have taken the time to discuss how they deliver care, adopted an existing guideline from a professional society or other organization or agreed on what the best practices are, and implemented them as the office's routine. Again, this signals commitment to providing consistently high-quality care and not allowing the kind of unjustified variation in care experienced by Ms. Wolf and her children at one of Washington, DC's, finest pediatric practices (page 87).

For patients like Mrs. Rodriguez (pages 93–94), who have chronic conditions—or family members finding a physician for a relative with chronic conditions—the fundamental question is whether the practice has embedded chronic care coordinators similar to those found at the Donna Medical Clinic or Iora Health (pages 99–100). For patients with serious chronic conditions, having a care coordinator who is co-located with the primary care or specialist physician is an absolute requirement. Indeed, if my father or mother had several chronic conditions, I would insist they go to a physician with care coordinators. It is the best way to ensure they get continuous attention and help staying on their care plan so they do not end up in the emergency room or admitted to the hospital.

Getting a practice that emphasizes effective care for behavioral and mental health issues is tricky. Ideally, all primary care and specialty practices would routinely screen patients for depression, anxiety disorders, and substance abuse and would have some form of collaborative care arrangement, either with co-located behavioral health specialists the way Dr. Nagoshi's Central Medical Clinic does (pages 138–139) or with a Quartet-like program to coordinate and expedite referrals from primary care providers to behavioral health specialists (pages 140–144). But that is not the world we live in today. So patients—or their relatives—need to be more selective. For patients who have or have had bouts of depression or baseline anxiety, it is probably absolutely necessary to ask whether the practice has some form of collaborative care arrangement. Conversely, for patients who do not have any current behavioral health issues, it is probably worth inquiring about the practice's behavioral health arrangements but not making it a requirement.

For patients with potentially life-threatening illnesses, such as cancer, congestive heart failure, or liver cirrhosis, or patients who are just elderly and very frail, it is important to be cared for the way Mrs. Winston is by Aspire (pages 145–146). As a patient or, more commonly, the family member of a patient with a potentially life-threatening illness, you want care providers to be coming to the home well before the last few days or weeks of life. It is important—indeed, necessary—to have visiting nurse practitioners who can address distressing symptoms such as pain, insomnia, diarrhea, constipation, and shortness of breath in the patient's home and coordinate all the caregivers so the patient does not have to repeatedly travel to a physician's office or hospital. Thus, it is important to ask whether the practice works with an agency that provides palliative care on the model of Aspire and not just hospice care right before death.

Similarly, for lower-income patients who need more social support and help navigating the health system, having an effective community healthcare worker program is definitely important and probably necessary to ensure high-value care. Patients like Lucas Downs (pages 151–152) need empathetic community health workers like Cheryl Garfield to help them get housing, select a compassionate primary care physician, and begin re-engaging socially by going to the mall, bowling, or to the movies, or finding them a wheelchair basketball league to play in. This will focus them on improving their lives and reduce their use of emergency rooms, readmissions, and other unnecessary interactions with the healthcare system.

Finally, for frail elderly and other patients at high risk of falling, few practices will have as extensive an exercise arrangement as Nifty after Fifty (pages 158–161, 220). But it is worth inquiring whether the medical practice has any exercise or lifestyle interventions to improve the patient's balance and strength and reduce the risk of falls. This is important but would not qualify as a necessary requirement for selecting a practice.

SHOULD I GET A CONCIERGE PHYSICIAN?

I do not recommend that people get a concierge physician. Concierge medicine has many allures, primarily access and time. For a fee, concierge practices ensure patients have immediate access to their physician through the phone and text messaging. They can also schedule same-day appointments with their physician and know that such visits won't be rushed, unlike what many patients experience at the average practice. All of this is appealing, especially for well-off Americans who have become used to not being part of the crowd and receiving personal, and even pampered, attention from companies.

From a system perspective, concierge medicine is not—and cannot—be transformative. Concierge medicine is just too small a market segment to be an important force in catalyzing a high-value delivery system. Some experts have estimated that there are just 5,000 concierge physicians in the United States. A recent survey of 19,000 physicians by WebMD reported that only 3% characterized themselves as concierge physicians. If these physicians care for small panels of patients to give each more time, then at most 5 million Americans are currently receiving concierge care. That makes it a niche market, catering to the 1%. This can hardly be considered a powerful force for change in American medicine. And it leaves the rest of us out.

But even from the patient's perspective, concierge medicine, while appealing for its access, is not optimal for its care. Every physician practice should offer open-access scheduling so patients can be seen the very day they call. As I have argued, this should not be limited to practices that charge an extra fee. But immediate access to physicians anytime you want on the phone or by text messaging? This availability may sound good to some people but is ultimately both undesirable and unnecessary. If patients really could call right to their physician, as if they were the physician's spouse, it would be terribly inefficient. As Simeon Schwartz of WESTMED says,

> Synchronous communication is extraordinarily expensive and inefficient. So if every patient has the doctor's cell phone numbers, what's the chance the doctor is going to see any patients and do any work? We do everything possible NOT to give the patients an opportunity to pick up the phone and reach the doctors directly.

Patients have a right to expect prompt access, but at transformed practices this is done asynchronously. Someone other than the physician interacts with the patient, managing their concerns using well-worked-out, standardized guidelines for common problems and, if the situation is more urgent, triaging the call. This is how John Sprandio's oncology group manages patient communication (pages 195–197).

Indeed, this is what most transformed practices do. For many groups, this type of communication has been very successful—and perhaps not surprisingly so. As Dr. Sprandio explains:

> We have efficient asynchronous communication, and that makes patients feel attended to and happy. So if we take Americans today, increasingly . . . they communicate with their friends when you're not with them by texting or things of that sort. You're not using their cell phone number to call them and have immediate access.

Although immediate access may feel good, concierge physicians are typically not able to offer many other aspects of transformed care. They do not necessarily engage in performance measurement and systematic efforts to rigorously evaluate and improve their practices in accordance with national benchmarks. Concierge physicians are typically selected by patients because of their reputation, not their documented outstanding performance. And their financial incentive is linked to the personal touch. Attentive, personal care is lovely and desirable, but it should not be confused with high-quality care. Although its patient-centric character is one facet of high-quality care, other aspects, such as surpassing national benchmarks on objective quality measures, are not integral to the concierge medicine model. When I emailed or called around to various high-end concierge practices or groups that manage concierge physicians to ask about whether they were recognized by NCQA as Patient Centered Medical Homes, we heard nothing. Other less-high-end practices that care for patients based on a monthly flat fee, so-called direct primary care practices, were a bit better. For instance, one, Direct Primary Care Coalition, reported that of their 59 physician practices, 3 are NCQA-certified PCMHs. Furthermore, the financial incentive in the upfront or monthly fee is not aligned with engaging in performance measurement, reporting, and improvement.

Concierge physicians tend to be organized into small practices. This means they typically lack the resources to add the other transformed practices. They do not necessarily have care managers for chronic conditions co-located in their offices or behavioral health specialists integrated right into their practices. Additionally, they often do not go through a process of standardizing their care; indeed, the ethos of concierge medicine is anti-standardization. Its philosophy is to treat every patient individually and personally. But that tailoring is often at odds with following the best-available research on optimal care and the evidence that standardized care delivers much more consistent, high-quality care. Concierge practices also tend to not have any organized way of delivering palliative care, such as contracts with companies like Aspire or other providers.

Instead, I recommend that patients follow the questions delineated here to choose their physicians (see Tables 9.2 and 9.3, pages 235 and 236). Many non-concierge practices can provide the access offered by concierge medicine through open-access scheduling and asynchronous communication. These practices are arguably more desirable, as they also have the potential to implement the 12 transformational practices. These medical organizations are truly dedicated to delivering high-quality care based on objective data and performance measurements. That is much better than concierge medicine.

AS THE PREVIOUS CHAPTERS make clear, the order in which practices prioritize transformational practices will not be the same as patients' individual priorities. The reason for this distinction is that patients are searching for a physician who can address their particular needs. Most Americans are relatively healthy or, at most, have just a few minor health problems. They, therefore, need a physician who has flexible scheduling and is very good at preventive care and managing common problems such as high cholesterol. For these patients, the key to selecting a physician is open-access scheduling and physicians dedication to performance improvement. Conversely, physicians are trying to transform their practices and are focused on improving the care they provide to thousands of patients, but especially high-risk, high-cost chronically ill patients who need the most attention and services. For physicians, the top priorities are chronic care coordination, open-access scheduling, performance measurement and improvement, and site of service. Although site of service is not typically what patients should worry about, it is of great concern to physicians trying to realize high-value care. Fortunately, there is enough overlap to ensure that physician practices engaged in transformation are precisely the practices patients should be selecting.

The questions posed here are simple, straightforward, and the best way for patients or their relatives to identify the right practice (see Tables 9.2 and 9.3, pages 235, 236). They certainly beat simply looking at glossy magazine rankings based on physician opinion without paying any systematic attention to whether those physicians have implemented the practices that ensure high-quality care. I do not suggest that this is an exhaustive checklist that will help you find the perfect physician, but I believe it is a good place to start. Had Miss Harris been equipped with these tools from the beginning, perhaps she would not currently be beholden to a bevy of healthcare providers, all working toward different goals. Our system is transforming—and for the better—but it will be years before that transformation ensures that all Americans receive high-quality lower-cost care. Until then, I hope this book can help guide patients through the changing healthcare landscape and allow them to receive the high-value care we all deserve.

ACKNOWLEDGMENTS

Honestly, I am not sure how this book began. To my best recollection my former Harvard Medical School classmate, colleague, and dear friend Harlan Krumholz of Yale is at least partially to blame. A long time ago he suggested that we could learn a lot by looking at health systems that were "positive outliers." At the time I did not give the idea much credence, but the notion of positive outliers stuck with me and rattled around in my brain. Then I began hearing about positive outliers among medical organizations that were doing great, transformative work, keeping chronically ill patients out of the hospital and improving care while also reducing costs. Arnie Milstein of Stanford mentioned CareMore to me. I met Craig Samitt, who was then working at Dean Clinic, and he told me about some of their important transformational practices. Andy Slavitt, when he was at Optum, mentioned that I needed to talk with Simeon Schwartz of WESTMED. Soon enough, a book idea about positive outliers who were transforming care in ways other physician practices and health systems could learn from began to take shape. I have to thank Simeon Schwartz in particular, because in the summer of 2016 his enthusiasm, insights, and all-around hutzpah persuaded me that I had all I needed to start writing and push along the transformational process. It was after our meeting that I took pen to paper—or, more accurately, fingers to computer keyboard.

This book could not have been researched and written without the extraordinary help from all those physicians, nurses, executives, and others at the various sites I visited who all devoted time to talking with me, delineating their programs, and correcting my mistakes about their organization. I have listed later in the acknowledgments the most important contributors and apologize to anyone I have failed to mention.

I need to thank Dave Johnson of 4Sight Health, who helped identify important sites that are delivering transformed care, accompanied me on many site visits, and provided extremely useful comments on drafts of this book.

In addition to Dave, Henry Aaron, Bob Kocher, and Eliza Barclay read drafts of numerous chapters and provided invaluable comments. They improved the text greatly, and despite their great efforts, the remaining flaws are not their responsibility. Special among my readers is my toughest critic and strictest editor, my daughter Natalia Emanuel—she spares nothing in critiquing my work. It is certainly all the better for her incisive comments and suggestions.

Through some magic I know not what, my assistant, Harlan Rosen, made time for me to write when there was no available time on the schedule. In no small measure his scheduling prowess actually made this book appear.

Teasel Muir-Harmony inspired me to finish the writing and editing, and made sure I stayed sitting at my desk while she took care of the necessary practicalities.

My literary agents Suzanne Gluck and Jennifer Randolph Walsh at WME have always given me sage advice about my book projects and helped shepherd this book to its conclusion.

Clive Priddle, Susan Weinberg, and Jaimie Leifer at PublicAffairs have now published and promoted 3 of my books. They are beyond wonderful to work with. They always remind me to keep the reader and the American public in mind. That advice, in addition to insightful comments, many precise edits, and everything else great publishers do, has made this both a better and more appealing book. Most of all I want to thank them for their faith in me and my work; they were willing to announce a book with very few words having been written.

My great appreciation goes to Andrew Steinmetz, Katie Chockley, Emily Gudbranson, Aaron Glickman, and John Urwin, my research assistants over the last 4 years. For many long hours they helped in numerous ways, from doing background research on the various sites to asking penetrating questions, from keeping transcripts to reading over and correcting multiple drafts. They did just about anything necessary to make this book successful. I cannot thank them enough because they always make me look better than I am.

PRESCRIPTION FOR THE FUTURE ACKNOWLEDGMENTS

From Advocate Health Care
  Lee Sacks
  Pankaj Patel
  Jeannine Herbst
  Dave Kemp

From Dean Clinic
  Allison Mooney
  Mark Kaufman

From Certify
  Marc Potash

From Quartet Health
  David Wennberg
  Marissa Bass

From Hoag Orthopedic Institute
  Alan Beyer
  James Caillouette
  Robert Gorab

From Aspire Health
  McKenzie
  Brad Smith

From Central Medical Clinic
  Mike Nagoshi

From VillageMD
  Tim Barry
  Clive Fields

From Blue Cross Blue Shield of Massachusetts
  Dana Gelb Safran

From Aledade
  Farzad Mostashari
  Adam Beckman

From the National Committee for Quality Assurance
Michael Barr
Margaret (Peggy) O'Kane

From Kaiser Permanente Mid-Atlantic
Bernadette Loftus
Greg Buehler
Susan Fiorella

From Group Health
Ira Segal
Scott Armstrong

From the Penn Center for Community Health Workers
Shreya Kangovia
Jill Feldstein
Cheryl Garfield

From Rio Grande Valley Accountable Care Organization (RGV ACO)
Jose Pena

From Iora Health
Andrew Schutzbank

From CareMore:
Leeba Lessin
Sachin Jain
Sheldon Zinberg

From WESTMED Medical Group
Simeon Schwartz

From ChenMed
James Chen
Chris Chen

APPENDIX

Tables and Figures

Table 2.1 Nine Provisions of the ACA Encouraging Payment and Delivery System Transformation

Provision	ACA section	Beginning date	Description
ACO	3022	December 2011	A network of physicians and other providers who coordinate care for a population of patients. Focuses on providing high-quality, evidence-based primary care. Shared savings for reducing costs below a government preset target. Voluntary Medicare demonstration project.
Medicare bundled payments	3023		Bundled payments are one price paid for all the services—physician fees, hospital care, rehabilitative services, home care, and so on—related to a discrete episode of care such as a hip replacement. Medicare is supposed to operate 5 voluntary pilot programs.
Center for Medicare and Medicaid Innovation (CMMI)	3021	January 1, 2011	Authority to conduct demonstration projects, including mandatory demonstration projects where physicians, hospitals, and other providers would have to participate. Budget of $10 billion.
Authorizing implementation of successful demonstration projects without additional legislation	3021	March 23, 2010	The secretary of HHS has the authority to implement payment changes as a permanent Medicare policy without the need for legislation based on any demonstration project that the Actuary certifies reduces costs without compromising quality, improves quality at no additional cost, or improves quality and reduces cost.

Hospital readmission policy	3025	October 1, 2012	Permanent change in policy to penalize hospitals with high rates of readmission within 30-days of Medicare patients for conditions such as acute myocardial infarctions.
Hospital-acquired conditions program	3008	October 1, 2014	Permanent change in policy to penalize hospitals that do not lower 14 hospital-acquired conditions such as ventilator-associated infections and medication errors.
Hospital value-based purchasing program	3001	October 1, 2012	Permanent change in policy to reward hospitals with bonus payments based on quality measures.
Patient Centered Outcomes Research Institute (PCORI)	6301	September 2010	Supports analysis of treatment, prevention, and diagnostic options; healthcare systems; health disparities; and patient-centered research. Helps disseminate findings. Expires in 2019.
Independent Payment Advisory Board (IPAB)	3403	2010*	Recommends policy changes to control healthcare spending if growth in per person Medicare costs exceeds 1% in 2017. Congress must either enact IPAB proposals or counter with other options.

*The members of the IPAB were supposed to be nominated by the President and confirmed by the Senate. No members have ever been nominated.

Table 2.2 Three Main Types of Medicare Accountable Care Organization Programs (ACOs)*

Type of ACO	Description	Result so far
Medicare Shared Savings Program (MSSP)	Physician-led organizations of at least 5,000 Medicare beneficiaries. Based on FFS payments. ACOs share in savings that are more than 2% below a government preset target benchmark budget.	433 ACOs with generally modest savings. In the most recent performance year about half the ACOs kept costs below the preset target benchmark and 31% kept costs below the threshold to share in savings. Quality metrics improved on average for nearly all ACOs.
Pioneer	Similar to MSSP, with financial responsibility for losses but also higher rewards for savings.	Began with 32 ACOs that have been reduced to 9. Significant improvement in quality scores with only about half sharing in savings
Next Generation	Graduation to capitated payment, higher risk and reward than the Pioneer and MSSP Programs.	Program begins in 2017.

*There is a fourth type of ACO program, the Advanced Payment ACO model, which essentially is the MSSP program for rural providers who receive up front charges.

Table 2.3 Four Major Bundled-Payment Initiatives

Program	Description	Mandatory or voluntary	Start date	Number of participants
Bundled Payment for Care Improvement—BPCI	4 models of episode payment for inpatient hospital services and post-acute services. Major bundles were for hip and knee replacement, congestive heart failure, and chronic obstructive pulmonary disease.	Voluntary	April 2013 (Model 1) October 2013 (Models 2, 3, and 4)	Model 1—1 Model 2—649 Model 3—862 Model 4—10
Comprehensive Care for Joint Replacement—CJR	Episode payment including in-hospital hip and knee replacement services, including physician fees, and 90 days post-hospital care. In August 2016 CMS expanded this bundle to include hip and femur fractures.	Mandatory	January 2016	67 geographic areas including nearly 800 hospitals
Oncology Care Model—OCM	6-month episode payments triggered by a start of chemotherapy, including fee-for-service payments, plus 2 bonus payments: (1) a $160 per-member per-month payment for coordinating care and (2) performance payments linked to quality and reductions in the patient's total cost of care.	Voluntary	July 1, 2016	194 oncology practices and 16 commercial payers

(continues)

Table 2.3 (*continued*)

Program	Description	Mandatory or voluntary	Start date	Number of participants
Cardiac bundles	Cover both CABG and AMI.* Bundled payment covers in-hospital services, physician services, and 90 days after discharge. CMS sets a target benchmark price that is adjusted for quality. Hospitals that save money and demonstrate high quality receive bonuses, and hospitals that exceed the target price must pay the money back.	Mandatory	July 2017	98 geographic areas (yet to be determined)

*CABG: coronary artery bypass graft surgery; AMI: acute myocardial infarction.

Table 2.4 The Language of Transformation

Phrase	Definition
Triple aim	First delineated in a 2008 article that claims the healthcare system should aim to simultaneously optimize 3 goals: (1) improving the health of the population, (2) reducing per capita costs, and (3) improving the patient experience of care.
Value-based payment	A strategy by payers to increase value by either improving healthcare quality or reducing costs or doing both. Models of value-based payment include ACO payments, pay for performance, and bundled payments.
Alternative payment model	CMS uses this phrase to describe any payment other than fee-for-service that will qualify for the goal of having 50% of CMS payments off fee-for-service by 2018. These include bundled-payment arrangements and ACO payments that include shared savings.
Capitation	A fixed per-patient payment, typically to a primary care provider to cover all of that provider's services for the patient, including office visits, case managers, and behavioral health services.
Value-based care	This is medical care that is designed in response to value-based payments to lead to measurable improvement in healthcare quality and reduced costs.
Patient-centric care	This is care designed to enhance the patient's experience by being sensitive to the patient's wants, needs, preferences, and educational requirements. Typically it focuses on 6 core elements: (1) education and shared knowledge, (2) involvement of family and friends, (3) collaborative team care, (4) inclusion of spiritual and nonmedical aspects of care, (5) respect for patient preferences, and (6) open access to medical information for the patient.
Population health	This aims to improve the health outcomes not just of an individual patient but of a group of patients—the population. The population typically includes not just patients who show up at the physicians' office but also those who have yet to access the healthcare system. It also focuses not just on clinical interventions but also includes public health as well as environmental and other factors that influence health outcomes.

Table 3.1 Six Essential Elements for Transformation

Element	Description and example
Catalyzing crisis	A near-death experience that makes people in the organization believe change is less risky than continuing on the same path.
	In 2008 Kaiser Permanente Mid-Atlantic had a near-death experience with declining membership, poor reputation, and declining and minimal margins based on underinvesting. It was going to be closed. Instead, it was taken over by Northern California Kaiser Permanente Medical Group and turned around.
Leadership	Someone—or a team—who establishes the organization's new direction and strategy and prioritizes steps for implementation. Analytic skills are comprised of 9 minimal threshold requirements, but the key distinguishing skill is emotional intelligence.
	Sheldon Zinberg is a charismatic leader who generates numerous disruptive ideas. He founded CareMore in 1991, dedicated to providing coordinated care for frail elderly patients. He also spearheaded the creation of exercise facilities—Nifty after Fifty—near the medical offices to integrate individually tailored exercise and prevention programs into care of seniors.
Culture, governance, and physician engagement	The ethos of an organization that employees implicitly or explicitly revert to for guidance on their jobs. It is composed of 6 aspects: vision, values, practices, people, narrative, and place.
	WESTMED empowers its physicians to ensure top-quality practice by having them develop their own practice guidelines and algorithms for managing common conditions, such as atrial fibrillation, and holds them accountable to their performance. It also consciously created waiting rooms with "Zen-like" visual and auditory experience by having TV screens showing calming nature photographs and having the spaces be quiet.

Element	Description and example
Data	All medical organizations need at least 5 types of data to transform: (1) claims data, (2) laboratory data, (3) imaging data, (4) pharmacy data, and (5) clinical data on hospital admissions data. The data are critical to identifying quality gaps, where the costs and excessive costs are, and performance of the physicians and other providers.
	Advocate Health Care has staff regularly visit physicians and review their current claims to review their performance compared to other physicians and national benchmarks.
Physician-management alignment	Creating financial and performance alignment between clinicians and operations to obtain front-line input and operations capacity to ensure effective implementation of transformational practices.
	Dean Clinic creates explicit physician-management dyads, pairing physician-leaders such as a clinic site chief with the clinic manager. The manager has authority over financial, physical, IT, and human resources to change processes of care. The physician can help identify changes to improve quality or reduce costs.
Financial risk	Creating financial incentives, usually through risk contracts, that reward improving quality, lowering costs, and enhancing patient experience. This is usually through risk-bearing contracts but can also be through creative fee-for-service arrangements with gainsharing.
	Kaiser Permanente Mid-Atlantic is an integrated delivery system that bears full risk based on premium. Many other organizations bear financial risk by being—or having capitated arrangements with—Medicare Advantage plans.

Table 4.1 The Twelve Practices of Transformation

Practice in the patient care process	Key components of transformation	Method of cost savings or altering service use*
Scheduling	Centralize scheduling.	Decreases per-unit cost.
	Open access to scheduling: leave 20% to 50% of physician and nurse practitioner appointment slots unscheduled at the start of every day.	Decreases utilization of high-cost sites or care such as the ER.
Registration and rooming	Create electronic registration that includes all patient and insurance information to eliminate repeat completion of forms by hand.	Decreases per-unit cost. Increases utilization of recommended services.
	Electronically link patients and EHRs to identify gaps in recommended tests and treatments that should be addressed (care gaps).	
	Have medical assistants rather than nurses room patients.	
	Empower medical assistants to close care gaps while rooming patients.	
	Have medical assistants highlight care gaps and abnormal values—for example, high blood pressure or hemoglobin A1c measurements—for physicians to address.	
Performance measurement and reporting	Establish metrics—preferably outcome and cost metrics—in collaboration with and acceptable to physicians.	Decreases utilization.
	Obtain timely—ideally real-time data—on individual provider performance, and benchmark to national standards.	
	Provide performance results to physicians in a timely manner—not longer than quarterly.	
	Disclose identified physician performance data so all physicians can learn from top performers.	
	Link salary or bonuses to both high performance and to improvement.	
Standardization of care	Identify common issues, often with variation in care.	Decreases utilization.
	Identify professional society, governmental, or other guidelines.	

Practice in the patient care process	Key components of transformation	Method of cost savings or altering service use*
	Empower physicians to create the guidelines and specific orders they think are optimal.	
	Create standard order sets to implement the guidelines, allowing physicians and others to override them when appropriate.	
Chronic care coordination	Identify high-risk, high-cost patients by predictive analytics and provider identification.	Increases the utilization of recommended services, leading to a decrease in high-cost services.
	Co-locate chronic care managers with primary care and specialist—such as oncology or cardiology—physicians.	
	Create personal relationships between the care managers and high-risk, high-cost patients and their families.	
	Encourage frequent contacts from care managers to patients to ensure compliance with measures—measuring hemoglobin A1c or weight—medications and other interventions.	
Shared decision making	Use available decision aides for preference-sensitive conditions, such as hip replacement for osteoarthritis or stents for stable angina.	Decreases utilization.
Site of service	In larger groups or health systems create centers of excellence for specialty care.	Decreases per-unit cost.
	Selectively contract with hospitals and skilled nursing facilities (SNFs). Sign per diem contracts so that if patients are discharged earlier, there are cost savings.	
	Employ hospitalists and/or nurse practitioners to care for patients in hospitals and SNFs.	
	Reward hospitalists based on reduced length of stay and readmission rates.	
	Utilize cost to select service providers for episodic, standardized interactions, such as laboratory testing, imaging services, and colonoscopies.	
	Use quality-ranking of similar services to identify high-performing specialists, and then selectively contract with high-performing specialists.	

(continues)

Table 4.1 (*continued*)

Practice in the patient care process	Key components of transformation	Method of cost savings or altering service use*
De-institutionalization	Use chronic care managers and others to institute tertiary prevention and reduce ER visits and hospitalization.	Decreases utilization. Decreases per-unit cost.
	Employ hospitalists at hospitals, SNFs, and other facilities to rapidly discharge patients to SNFs or home.	
	Substitute home care for hospitalizations for patients with acute exacerbations of chronic conditions—such as congestive heart failure—or acute illnesses—like pneumonia or urinary tract infections.	
	Reduce readmissions by arranging for either a home visit or an office visit within 7 days of hospital discharge.	
Behavioral health interventions	Routinely screen all patients for depression and anxiety with standardized tools such as PHQ-9 and GAD-7.	Decreases utilization.
	Co-locate behavioral health specialists with primary care or specialist physicians in the same office.	
	Create personal relationships between the behavioral health specialists and patients or refer patients to a specialized behavioral health service that connects patients to specialists and oversees their care.	
Palliative care	Identify patients with a prognosis of 1 year or less through provider identification and predictive analytics.	Decreases utilization.
	Refer patients to specialized palliative care services that send palliative care specialists to routinely visit patients at home.	
Community interventions	Provide resources for daily life. Assist with health system navigation. Provide medical assistance, such as help obtaining medications.	Increases utilization of recommended services, leading to a decrease in high-cost services.
	Encourage lifestyle changes, such as exercising with patients at the YMCA.	
	Provide psychosocial support.	
	Hire for empathy to ensure providers are compassionate.	

Practice in the patient care process	Key components of transformation	Method of cost savings or altering service use*
Lifestyle interventions	Create organized and free exercise opportunities, initially for elderly patients, focusing on balance and strength to reduce falls and hip fractures.	Increases utilization of recommended services, leading to decrease in high-cost services.
	Expand opportunities to ensure patients exercise 30 minutes a day, 5 times a week.	
	Consider other lifestyle interventions such as providing vegetables, fruits, and other nutritious foods with cooking instructions to people with diabetes.	

*Total costs are a product of price times volume—that is, the cost per unit and utilization or number of services used. Thus, cost savings can be achieved either by improving efficiency and decreasing costs per unit or by decreasing unnecessary or even harmful numbers of units. Sometimes the goal actually is to increase utilization of certain services in order to reduce the use of more expensive services. Examples include getting diabetics to adhere to medications and lower their hemoglobin A1c's below 7%; adherence to medications to reduce blood pressure and cholesterol; taking aspirin; and quitting or reducing smoking—all of which should result in fewer hospital admissions for a variety of diabetic side effects such as renal failure, heart attacks, infections, and amputations. Therefore, increases in some services and medications may lead to reductions in other, typically more costly services.

Table 4.2 Five Steps in Managing Patients with Chronic Illnesses

Steps	Description	Example
Identify high-risk patients.	Use data and "medical intuition" to identify patients who are high-cost, unstable, or likely to be hospitalized.	Iora's worry score, which has 4 levels: emergent, high, medium, and low worry. Attention is devoted to 8% to 9% of high-risk patients where the trajectory of care can be changed with care management.
Embed care managers in primary and specialty care teams.	Physically co-locate chronic care coordinators with the care teams.	VillageMD has the physician personally introduce the care manager to the patient and family in the exam room to create a personal bond.
Empower care coordinators or others in the office to close care gaps.	Do not rely on physicians to close care gaps; instead, entrust closing care gaps to care coordinators or others in the clinic.	Have care managers or rooming medical assistants order standard tests and procedures, such as flu shots and colonoscopies.
Provide high-touch care.	Contact high-cost, high-risk patients by phone, see them at special clinics—for example, nutrition counseling—or conduct frequent home visits.	Donna Medical Clinic has the care coordinators calling patients weekly to check in on the key physiological risk factors and on medication compliance and coming to the office. Unstable patients have regular home visits by nurse practitioner.
Realize aims of frequent contacts	(1) Educate about the patient's disease. (2) Encourage disease monitoring. (3) Promote medication compliance. (4) Create social engagement. (5) Train patients to call or come to the office rather than the emergency room.	CareMore constantly educates its diabetic patients about their disease, the importance of eating right, coming to get their toenails clipped to avoid cuts, measuring their glucose, and taking their insulin. It educates them in the office, on the phone, and during meetings with a dietician or a toenail clipping session. It creates frequent interactions and uses everyone to educate and promote adherence to the treatment plan.

Figure 4.1 Blinded Comparison of Emergency Room Discharge Time by Provider

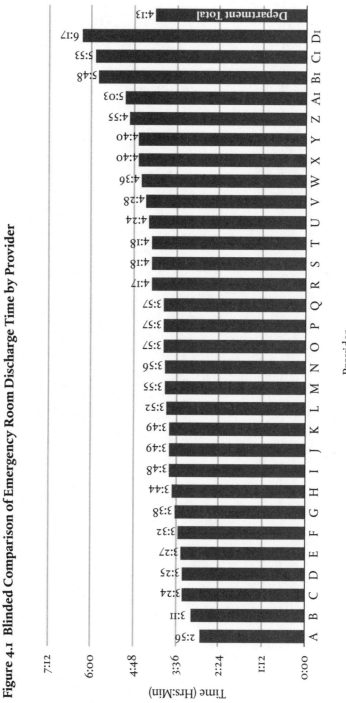

Provider	Time (Hrs:Min)
A	2:56
B	3:11
C	3:24
D	3:25
E	3:27
F	3:32
G	3:38
H	3:44
I	3:48
J	3:49
K	3:49
L	3:52
M	3:55
N	3:56
O	3:57
P	3:57
Q	3:57
R	4:17
S	4:18
T	4:18
U	4:24
V	4:28
W	4:36
X	4:40
Y	4:40
Z	4:55
A1	5:03
B1	5:48
C1	5:53
D1	6:17
Department Total	4:13

Figure 4.2 Expenditures by Patient Group, 2011

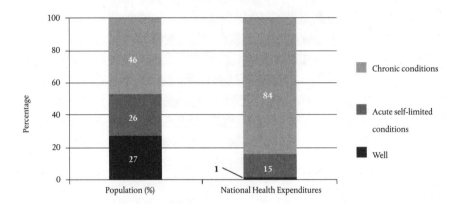

Source: http://jamanetwork.com/journals/jama/fullarticle/176989

Figure 4.3 Distribution of Health Expenditures in the United States, 2010

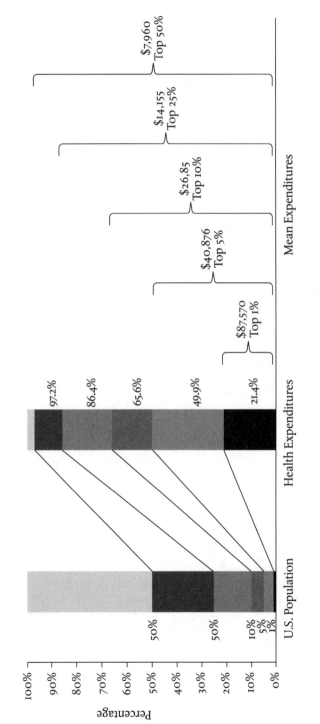

Source: Center for Financing, Access, and Cost Trends, AHRQ, Household Component of the Medical Expenditure Panel Survey, 2010

Table 5.1 Steps for Implementing Shared Decision Making

Step	Explanation
Provider training	Have clinicians watch the decision aide video or read decision aide material. Train clinicians on how to talk to patients to elicit their preferences.
Integration into workflow	Have the PCP provide patients the decision aide prior to seeing specialists or making a decision.
"Feed-forward" patient assessment	After the patients have viewed or read the decision aide, they should complete a survey assessing knowledge and preferences. Provide the results to the clinician.
Tracking and reporting on decision aide use and utilization of preference-sensitive conditions	Provide clinicians with unblinded comparative data on the frequency of decision aide use and with the utilization of the medical procedure.

Table 6.1 Five Core Functions of Community Healthcare Workers

Domain	Example
Resources for daily life	Collect or obtain birth certificates, social security cards, and utility bills to obtain driver's licenses or other state IDs.
	Help apply for housing, daycare, food stamps, home ramps, and other social services.
Health system navigation	Help apply for health insurance.
	Find a suitable primary care physician.
	Help schedule and travel to appointments.
	Obtain health records from myriad health systems.
Medical assistance	Help obtain medications and durable medical equipment.
	Coach patients prior to an appointment about what to ask and get information in a way they can understand.
	Encourage patients to write down questions to ask physicians during an appointment.
	Accompany patients to grief or addiction counseling.
Lifestyle change	Exercise with patients at YMCA.
	Encourage patients to start a weight-loss contest or attend smoking-cessation classes.
Psychosocial support	Take the patients to enjoyable activities, such as bowling, fishing, or the movies.
	Help patients sign up for community volunteer activities.

Table 6.2 Six Keys to Success of Community Healthcare Work Programs

Activity	Examples
Hiring	Hire for listening skills and human connectedness—compassion, empathy, engagement.
	Hire community organizers, social service personnel, and customer service workers.
	De-emphasize academic credentials.
Training	Train for all levels of employment: program directors, managers, and community health workers.
	Base 1-month community health worker training on adult learning theory, such as role playing.
	Spend 2 weeks shadowing a senior community health worker and 2 weeks being shadowed by a senior community health worker.
Standardized interviewing	Use semistructured interview techniques based on social science theory.
Safety	Community health workers meet their clients individually only in public places. If they go to the patients' houses, they go with colleagues. Managers call workers 30 minutes into a solo visit and after 60 minutes in a 2-staff member visit.
	Safety huddles involving manager and director to identify and address safety concerns.
Data	Data coordinators who systematically track outcomes and provide performance reports.
Supervision and management	Weekly meeting between project manager and each community worker to ensure:
	• Realistic goals, plan of care, and timeline • Progress on meeting goals • Overcoming obstacles • Debrief for stress reduction

Table 8.1 The Tiering of Transformation

Tier 1	Tier 2	Tier 3
Scheduling	Registration and rooming	Shared decision making
Performance measurement	Standardization	Palliative care
Chronic care coordination	De-institutionalization	Community health workers
Site of service	Behavioral and mental healthcare	Lifestyle interventions

Table 9.1 How the Transformational Practices Can Help Patients Pick a Physician

Absolutely necessary	*Important for select types of patients*	*Nice to have*
Scheduling Must have open-access scheduling.	**Standardization** For all patients, a practice should develop and use standardized treatment pathways or protocols for common conditions.	**Registration and rooming** Would be desirable to have electronic registration with Certify or other RFID-enabled technology.
Performance measurement Must participate in some kind of standardized assessment of performance in comparison to local and national benchmarks such as NCQA.	**Chronic care management** For patients with chronic illnesses, practices should use a care manager or coordinator co-located in the practice.	**Shared decision making** For patients with a condition that has preference-sensitive interventions, such as hip replacement, or chronic chest pain, use decision aides to educate patients.
	De-institutionalization For patients with chronic conditions that cause frequent hospitalizations, such as congestive heart failure or emphysema or asthma, a practice should have arrangements for care at home.	**Site of service** Should have contracts with and refer patients to high-value specialists and high-quality hospitals.
	Behavioral and mental health Patients with a history of depression or anxiety should have some collaborative care arrangement either through co-location of a behavioral health specialist or use of a Quartet-like agency to coordinate behavioral health referrals. For other patients the practice should routinely screen for depression and anxiety and should have prompt access to behavioral health specialists.	**Lifestyle interventions** Patients at high risk for certain problems such as falls should have access to balance and strength-training programs.

Absolutely necessary	Important for select types of patients	Nice to have
	Home and palliative care For patients with limited (roughly one year) life expectancy, such as those with advanced cancer or end-stage congestive heart failure, a practice should have not just hospice but also home-based palliative care services available months before anticipated end of life.	
	Community healthcare workers For patients with few social supports, a practice should have community healthcare workers who can facilitate social services and social engagement.	

Table 9.2 Two Absolutely Necessary Questions to Ask when Selecting a Physician

Initial question	Potential follow-up question
Does your practice have open-access scheduling?	If yes, then ask: What proportion of appointment slots are left unscheduled each day?
Is your practice an NCQA-recognized Patient Centered Medical Home (PCMH)?	If no, then ask: Does the practice participate in any systematic performance measurement and improvement activity similar to NCQA assessments?

Table 9.3 Important Questions to Ask when Selecting a Physician for Patients with Particular Conditions

Type of patient	Type of question
For all patients	Does the practice have standardized pathways or protocols the physicians follow for common conditions such as:
	For children: ear infections, asthma, upper-respiratory infections?
	For adults: high blood pressure, high cholesterol, asthma, or blood thinning?
For patients with chronic conditions such as congestive heart failure, diabetes, or emphysema	Does the practice have a chronic care coordinator located in the office who helps manage patients with chronic illnesses?
For patients with life-threatening conditions such as metastatic cancer, end-stage congestive heart failure, or liver cirrhosis.	Does the practice work with an agency to provide palliative care—not hospice care—at home?
For lower-income patients lacking social supports	Does the practice have community healthcare workers who help patients who need more social services and social engagement?

FURTHER READING

CHAPTER 1. FAILING MISS HARRIS

DeJonge, K. E., G. Taler, and P. A. Boling. "Independence at Home: Community-Based Care for Older Adults with Severe Chronic Illness." *Clinics in Geriatric Medicine* 25, no. 1 (February 2009): 155–69.

Esposito, L. "Defibrillator Insertion: Implant for Life." *US News & World Report*, November 26, 2014. http://health.usnews.com/health-news/patient-advice/articles/2014/11/26/defibrillator-insertion-implant-for-life.

Morrison, R. S., J. Dietrich, S. Ladwig et al. "Palliative Care Consultation Teams Cut Hospital Costs for Medicaid Beneficiaries." *Health Affairs* 30, no. 3 (March 2011): 454–63. doi:10.1377/hlthaff.2010.0929.

Neuman, P., J. Cubanski, and A. Damico. "Medicare Per Capita Spending by Age and Service: New Data Highlights Oldest Beneficiaries." *Health Affairs* 34, no. 2 (February 2015): 335–39. doi:10.1377/hlthaff.2014.1371.

Teno, J. M., P. L. Gozalo, J. P. W. Bynum et al. "Change in End-of-Life Care for Medicare Beneficiaries: Site of Death, Place of Care, and Health Care Transitions in 2000, 2005, and 2009." *Journal of the American Medical Association* 309, no. 5 (February 2013): 470–77. doi:10.1001/jama.2012.207624.

CHAPTER 2. THE STIMULUS FOR CHANGE:
ACA, BUNDLED PAYMENTS, MACRA, AND BEYOND

American Hospital Associations. "Medicare's Bundled Payment Initiatives: Considerations for Providers." January 19, 2016. www.aha.org/content/16/iss brief-bundledpmt.pdf.

Emanuel, E. J. "How Well Is the Affordable Care Act Doing? Reasons for Optimism." *Journal of the American Medical Association* 315, no. 13 (April 2016): 1331–32. http://jamanetwork.com/journals/jama/fullarticle/2499847.

Emanuel, E. J. *Reinventing American Health Care*. New York: Public Affairs, 2014.

Emanuel, E. J., and R. Kocher. "Republican Criticisms of Obamacare Are Extremely Misleading." *Vox*, October 19, 2016. www.vox.com/the-big-idea/2016/10/19/13331498/republican-criticisms-obamacare-misleading.

Emanuel, E. J., and R. Kocher. "Yes, Obama Care Needs Tweaks—But It's Been a Policy Triumph." *Vox,* October 7, 2016. www.vox.com/the-big-idea/2016/10/7/13192640/obamacare-exchanges-insurance-healthcare-fix.

Emanuel, E. J., and T. Spiro. "The Affordable Care Act Is Not in Crisis—But It Could Be Better." *Washington Post,* August 22, 2016. www.washingtonpost.com/news/in-theory/wp/2016/08/22/the-affordable-care-act-is-not-in-crisis-but-it-could-be-better/?utm_term=.c668b4f6cceb.

Lewin Group. "CMS Bundled Payments for Care Improvement Initiative Models 2–4: Year 2 Evaluation and Monitoring Annual Report." 2016. https://innovation.cms.gov/Files/reports/bpci-models2-4-yr2evalrpt.pdf.

Skinner, J., and A. Chandra. "The Past and Future of the Affordable Care Act." *Journal of the American Medical Association* 316, no 5 (August 2016): 497. http://jamanetwork.com/journals/jama/fullarticle/2533697.

Zuckerman, R. B., S. H. Sheingold, E. J. Orav et al. "Readmissions, Observation, and the Hospital Readmissions Reduction Program." *NEJM* 374, no. 16 (April 2016). www.nejm.org/doi/full/10.1056/NEJMsa1513024?source=acsh.org#t=article.

CHAPTER 3. SIX ESSENTIAL ELEMENTS
OF TRANSFORMATION

"2017 Star Ratings." CMS. www.cms.gov/Newsroom/MediaReleaseDatabase/Fact-sheets/2016-Fact-sheets-items/2016-10-12.html.

Britnell, M. "Transforming Health Care Takes Continuity and Consistency." *Harvard Business Review,* December 28, 2015. https://hbr.org/2015/12/transforming-health-care-takes-continuity-and-consistency.

Jha, A., and A. Epstein. "Hospital Governance and the Quality of Care." *Health Affairs* 29, no. 1 (January 2010): 182–87. http://content.healthaffairs.org/content/29/1/182.short.

Murdoch, T. B. and A. S. Detsky. "The Inevitable Application of Big Data to Health Care." *Journal of the American Medical Association* 309, no. 13 (2013): 1351. http://jamanetwork.com/journals/jama/fullarticle/1674245.

Porter, M. E. "What Is Value in Health Care?" *New England Journal of Medicine,* December 23, 2010. www.nejm.org/doi/full/10.1056/Nejmp1011024#t=article.

Suter, E., N. D. Oelke, C. E. Adair et al. "Ten Key Principles for Successful Health Systems Integration." *Healthcare Quarterly* 13(2009): 16–23. www.ncbi.nlm.nih.gov/pmc/articles/PMC3004930.

CHAPTER 4. THE 12 PRACTICES OF TRANSFORMATION: TRANSFORMING THE PHYSICIAN OFFICE INFRASTRUCTURE

Scheduling

Committee on Optimizing Scheduling in Health Care, Institute of Medicine, G. S. Kaplan et al., eds. "Transforming Health Care Scheduling and Access: Getting to Now." Washington, DC: National Academies Press. August 24, 2015. www.ncbi.nlm.nih.gov/books/NBK316141.

Kaplan, G. S. "Health Care Scheduling and Access Report from the IOM." *Journal of the American Medical Association* 314, no. 14 (October 2015):1449–50. doi:10.1001/jama.2015.9431.

Mehrotra, A., L. Keehl-Markowitz, and J. Z. Ayanian. "Implementation of Open Access Scheduling in Primary Care: A Cautionary Tale." *Annals of Internal Medicine* 148, no. 12 (2008): 915–22.

Performance Measurement

Cassel, C. K., and S. H. Jain. "Assessing Individual Physician Performance: Does Measurement Suppress Motivation?" *Journal of the American Medical Association* 307, no. 24 (2012): 2595–96. http://jamanetwork.com/journals/jama/full article/1199161.

Higgins, A., G. Veselovskiy, and L. McKown. "Provider Performance Measures in Private and Public Programs: Achieving Meaningful Alignment with Flexibility to Innovate." *Health Affairs* 32, no. 8 (August 2013): 1453–61. http://content.healthaffairs.org/content/32/8/1453.full.

Provonost, P. J., and R. Lilford. "A Road Map for Improving the Performance of Performance Measurement." *Health Affairs* 30, no. 4 (April 2011): 569–73. http://content.healthaffairs.org/content/30/4/569.full.

Roski, J., and M. McClellan. "Measuring Health Care Performance Now, Not Tomorrow: Essential Steps to Support Effective Health Reform." *Health Affairs* 30, no. 4 (April 2011): 682–89. http://content.healthaffairs.org/content/30/4/682.full.

Standardization

Porter, M. E., S. Larsson, and T. H. Lee. "Standardizing Patient Outcomes Measurement." *New England Journal of Medicine* 374, no. 6 (February 2016): 504–6. doi:10.1056/nejmp1511701.

Chronic Care Coordination

Aronson, L., C. A. Bautista, and K. Covinsky. "Medicare and Care Coordination: Expanding the Clinician's Toolbox." *Journal of the American Medical Association* 313, no. 8 (February 2015): 797–98. doi:10.1001/jama.2014.18174.

Bodenheimer, T., E. Chen, and H. D. Bennett. "Confronting the Growing Burden of Chronic Disease: Can the U.S. Health Care Workforce Do the Job?" *Health Affairs* 28, no. 1 (2009): 64–74. doi:10.1377/hlthaff.28.1.64.

Wiley, J. A., D. R. Rittenhouse, S. M. Shortell et al. "Managing Chronic Illness: Physician Practices Increased the Use of Care Management and Medical Home Processes." *Health Affairs* 34, no. 1 (May 2015): 78–86. doi:10.1377/hlthaff.2014.0404.

CHAPTER 5. THE TWELVE PRACTICES OF TRANSFORMATION: TRANSFORMING PROVIDER INTERACTIONS

Shared Decision Making

Arterburn, D., D. R. Flum, E. O. Westbrook et al. "A Population-Based, Shared Decision-Making Approach to Recruit for a Randomized Trial of Bariatrics Surgery Versus Lifestyle for Type 2 Diabetes." *Surgery for Obesity and Related Diseases* 9, no. 6 (November–December 2013): 837–44. doi:10.1016/j.soard.2013.05.006.

Arterburn, D., R. Wellman, E. Westbrook et al. "Introducing Decision Aids at Group Health Was Linked to Sharply Lower Hip and Knee Surgery Rates and Costs." *Health Affairs* 31, no. 9 (September 2012): 2094–2104. doi:10.1377/hlthaff.2011.0686.

Gillick, M. R. "Guiding the Guardians and Other Participants in Shared Decision Making." *Journal of the American Medical Association* 175, no. 10 (January 2015): 1691. http://jamanetwork.com/journals/jamainternalmedicine/fullarticle/2426424.

Hoffman, T. C., V. M. Montori, and C. Del Mar. "The Connection Between Evidence-Based Medicine and Shared Decision Making." *Journal of the American Medical Association* 312, no. 13 (October 2014): 1295–96. http://jamanetwork.com/journals/jama/fullarticle/1910118.

Kupperman, M., and G. F. Sawaya. "Shared Decision-Making: Easy to Evoke, Challenging to Implement." *Journal of the American Medical Association Internal Medicine* 175, no. 2 (February 2015): 167–68. http://jamanetwork.com/journals/jamainternalmedicine/fullarticle/1936575.

Lee, E. O., and E. J. Emanuel. "Shared Decision Making to Improve Care and Reduce Costs." *New England Journal of Medicine* 368, no. 1 (January 2013): 6–8. doi:10.1056/nejmp1209500.

Site of Service

Barnett, M. L., Z. Song, and B. E. Landon. "Trends in Physician Referrals in the United States, 1999–2009." *Archives of Internal Medicine* 172, no. 2 (January 2012): 163–170. doi:10.1001/archinternmed.2011.722.

Mostashari, F., and T. Broome. "The Opportunities and Challenges of the MSSP ACO Program: A Report from the Field." *American Journal of Managed Care* 22, no. 9 (September 2016): 564–68.

De-institutionalization

Cryer, L., S. B. Shannon, M. Van Amsterdam et al. "Costs for 'Hospital at Home' Patients Were 19 Percent Lower, with Equal or Better Outcomes Compared to Similar Patients." *Health Affairs* 31, no. 6 (June 2012): 1237–43. http://content .healthaffairs.org/content/31/6/1237.abstract.

Kinosian, B., G. Taler, P. Boling et al. "Projected Savings and Workforce Transformation from Converting Independence at Home to a Medicare Benefit." *Journal of the American Geriatrics Society* 64, no. 8 (August 2016): 1531–36. doi:10.1111/ jgs.14176.

Leff, B. "Why I Believe in Hospital at Home." *New England Journal of Medicine Catalyst*, February 5, 2016. http://catalyst.nejm.org/why-i-believe-in-hospital -at-home.

Marchica, J. "Reinventing Home Health." *Health Affairs Blog.* August 11, 2015. http:// healthaffairs.org/blog/2015/08/11/reinventing-home-health.

CHAPTER 6. THE TWELVE PRACTICES OF TRANSFORMATION: EXPANDING THE SCOPE OF CARE

Behavioral Health Interventions

Gilbody, S., P. Bower, J. Fletcher et al. "Collaborative Care for Depression: A Cumulative Meta-analysis and Review of Longer-Term Outcomes." *Archives of Internal Medicine* 166, no. 21 (November 2006): 2314–21. doi:10.1001/archinte.166.21.2314.

Katon, W. J., E. H. Lin, M. V. Korff et al. "Collaborative Care for Patients with Depression and Chronic Illnesses." *New England Journal of Medicine* 363, no. 27 (December 2010): 2611–20. doi:10.1056/nejmoa1003955.

Katon, W. J., M. Von Korff, E. H. B. Lin et al. "The Pathways Study: A Randomized Trial of Collaborative Care in Patients with Diabetes and Depression." *Archives of General Psychiatry* 61, no. 10 (2004): 1042–49. doi:10.1001/archpsyc.61.10.1042.

Simon, G. E., W. J. Katon, M. Vonkorff, et al. "Cost-Effectiveness of a Collaborative Care Program for Primary Care Patients with Persistent Depression." *American Journal of Psychiatry* 158, no. 10 (October 2001): 1638–44. doi:10.1176/appi .ajp.158.10.1638.

Home and Palliative Care

Kamal, A. H., K. L. Harrison, M. Bakitas et al. "Improving the Quality of Palliative Care Throughout National and Regional Collaboration Efforts." *Cancer Control* 22, no. 4 (October 2015): 396–402. https://moffitt.org/media/4654/396.pdf.

Community Interventions

Kangovi, S., N. Mitra, D. Grande et al. "Patient-Centered Community Health Worker Intervention to Improve Posthospital Outcomes: A Randomized Clinical Trial." *Journal of the American Medical Association Internal Medicine* 174, no. 4 (2014): 535–45. www.ncbi.nlm.nih.gov/pubmed/24515422.

CHAPTER 7. VIRTUAL MEDICINE: A RED HERRING?

Beck, M. "How Telemedicine Is Transforming Health Care." *Wall Street Journal*, June 26, 2016. www.wsj.com/articles/how-telemedicine-is-transforming -health-care-1466993402.

Finkelstein, E. A., B. A. Haaland, M. Bilger et al. "Effectiveness of Activity Trackers with and Without Incentives to Increase Physical Activity (TRIPPA): A Randomised Controlled Trial." *Lancet Diabetes and Endocrinology* 4, no. 12 (December 2016): 983–95.

Grabowsky, D. C., and A. J. O'Malley. "Use of Telemedicine Can Reduce Hospitalizations of Nursing Home Residents and Generate Savings for Medicare." *Health Affairs* 33, no. 2 (February 2013): 244–50. http://content.healthaffairs.org/content/33/2/244.abstract.

Greene, J. A. "Do-It-Yourself Medical Devices: Technology and Empowerment in American Health Care." *New England Journal of Medicine* 374, no. 4 (January 2016): 305–8. www.nejm.org/doi/full/10.1056/NEJMp1511363?af=R&rss=current Issue#t=article.

Kahn, J. M. "Virtual Visits—Confronting the Challenges of Telemedicine." *New England Journal of Medicine* 372, no. 18 (January 2015): 1684–85. www.nejm.org/doi/full/10.1056/NEJMp1500533.

Kvedar, J., M. J. Coye, and W. Everett. "Connected Health: A Review of Technologies and Strategies to Improve Patient Care with Telemedicine and Telehealth." *Health Affairs* 33, no 2 (February 2014): 194–99. http://content.healthaffairs.org/content/33/2/194.abstract.

Mehrotra, A., A. B. Jena, A. B. Busch et al. "Utilization of Telemedicine Among Rural Medicare Beneficiaries." *Journal of the American Medical Association* 315, no. 18 (May 2016): 2015–16. doi:10.1001/jama.2016.2186.

Obermeyer, Z., and E. J. Emanuel. "Predicting the Future—Big Data, Machine Learning, and Clinical Medicine." *New England Journal of Medicine* 375, no. 13 (September 2016): 1216–19. doi:10.1056/nejmp1606181.

Ong, M. K., P. S. Romano, S. Edgington et al. "Effectiveness of Remote Patient Monitoring After Discharge of Hospitalized Patients with Heart Failure: The Better Effectiveness After Transition–Heart Failure (BEAT-HF): Randomized Clinical Trial." *Journal of the American Medical Association Internal Medicine* 176, no. 3 (March 2016): 310–18. doi:10.1001/jamainternmed.2015.7712.

Patel, M. S., D. A. Asch, and K. G. Volpp. "Wearable Devices as Facilitators, Not Drivers, of Health Behavior Change." *Journal of the American Medical Association* 313, no. 5 (February 2015): 459–60.

Topol, E. J. *The Creative Destruction of Medicine: How the Digital Revolution Will Create Better Health Care*. New York: Basic Books, 2013.

CHAPTER 8.
IS TRANSFORMED HEALTHCARE TRANSFERABLE?

Collins, J. C. *Good to Great: Why Some Companies Make the Leap . . . And Others Don't*. New York: HarperBusiness, 2001.

Goldsmith, J., and L. Burns. "Fail to Scale: Why Great Ideas in Health Care Don't Thrive Everywhere." *Health Affairs Blog*, September 29, 2016. http://health affairs.org/blog/2016/09/29/fail-to-scale-why-great-ideas-in-health-care -dont-thrive-everywhere.

Kotter, J. P. *Leading Change*. Boston: Harvard Business School Press, 1996.

Kotter, J. P. "Leading Change: Why Transformation Efforts Fail." *Harvard Business Review* (January 2007). doi:10.1109/emr.2009.5235501.

Richard M. J., and M. B. Bohmer. "The Hard Work of Health Care Transformation." *New England Journal of Medicine* 375, no. 8 (August 2016): 709–11. www .nejm.org/doi/full/10.1056/NEJMp1606458#t=article.

INDEX

ABOUT THE AUTHOR

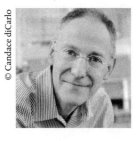

Ezekiel J. Emanuel is the vice provost for Global Initiatives, the Diane V. S. Levy and Robert M. Levy University Professor, and chair of the Department of Medical Ethics and Health Policy at the University of Pennsylvania. He is also a senior fellow at the Center for American Progress. Dr. Emanuel was the founding chair of the Department of Bioethics at the National Institutes of Health from January 2009 to August 2011. Until January 2011, he served as a special advisor on Health Policy to the Director of the Office of Management and Budget and the National Economic Council. He is a breast oncologist and author of several books, including *Healthcare, Guaranteed* and *Reinventing American Healthcare* (both PublicAffairs).

PublicAffairs is a publishing house founded in 1997. It is a tribute to the standards, values, and flair of three persons who have served as mentors to countless reporters, writers, editors, and book people of all kinds, including me.

I. F. STONE, proprietor of *I. F. Stone's Weekly*, combined a commitment to the First Amendment with entrepreneurial zeal and reporting skill and became one of the great independent journalists in American history. At the age of eighty, Izzy published *The Trial of Socrates*, which was a national bestseller. He wrote the book after he taught himself ancient Greek.

BENJAMIN C. BRADLEE was for nearly thirty years the charismatic editorial leader of *The Washington Post*. It was Ben who gave the *Post* the range and courage to pursue such historic issues as Watergate. He supported his reporters with a tenacity that made them fearless and it is no accident that so many became authors of influential, best-selling books.

ROBERT L. BERNSTEIN, the chief executive of Random House for more than a quarter century, guided one of the nation's premier publishing houses. Bob was personally responsible for many books of political dissent and argument that challenged tyranny around the globe. He is also the founder and longtime chair of Human Rights Watch, one of the most respected human rights organizations in the world.

·   ·   ·

For fifty years, the banner of Public Affairs Press was carried by its owner Morris B. Schnapper, who published Gandhi, Nasser, Toynbee, Truman, and about 1,500 other authors. In 1983, Schnapper was described by *The Washington Post* as "a redoubtable gadfly." His legacy will endure in the books to come.

Peter Osnos, *Founder and Editor-at-Large*